100 Questions & Answers About Myeloma

Asad Bashey, MD, PhD
*University of California,
San Diego*

James W. Huston

JONES AND BARTLETT PUBLISHERS
Sudbury, Massachusetts
BOSTON   TORONTO   LONDON   SINGAPORE

World Headquarters
Jones and Bartlett
Publishers
40 Tall Pine Drive
Sudbury, MA 01776
info@jbpub.com
www.jbpub.com

Jones and Bartlett
Publishers Canada
2406 Nikanna Road
Mississauga, ON L5C 2W6
CANADA

Jones and Bartlett
Publishers International
Barb House, Barb Mews
London W6 7PA
UK

Library of Congress Cataloging-in-Publication Data

Bashey, Asad, 1960-
  100 questions and answers about myeloma / Asad Bashey, James W. Hurston.— 1st ed.
    p. cm.
  Includes index.
  ISBN 0-7637-4553-7 (pbk. : alk. paper)
  1. Multiple myeloma—Popular works. I. Title: One hundred questions and answers about myeloma. II. Hurston, James W. III. Title.
  RC280.B6B376 2005
  616.99'418—dc22

                                                     2004020311

Production Credits
Executive Publisher: Christopher Davis
Production Manager: Amy Rose
Associate Production Editor: Renée Sekerak
Editorial Assistant: Kathy Richardson
Marketing Manager: Matthew Payne
Manufacturing Buyer: Therese Bräuer
Cover Design: Colleen Halloran
Composition: Northeast Compositors, Inc.
Printing and Binding: Malloy, Inc.
Cover Printing: Malloy, Inc.

Printed in the United States of America

08 07 06 05   10 9 8 7 6 5 4 3 2

Contents

This book is for patients with myeloma and their relatives and friends. It is written by a physician with extensive experience in treating and supporting myeloma patients and a patient who has experienced almost all the commonly available treatment options for this disease while pursuing a challenging career. By using a question and answer format and straightforward explanation of commonly encountered technical terms, this book is designed to help answer many of the questions and concerns encountered by myeloma patients and their friends and families. We hope this book can help you take an active role in your care and be more confident in discussing your illness and the treatment options available to you with your healthcare providers and other interested persons.

Encountering myeloma for the first time is a shock, whether you are the patient, a member of a patient's family, or a friend. You will learn it is a life-threatening disease, and will be need to understand and cope with the challenges of a disease you may not have known anything about previously. The physicians you encounter may talk about "electrophoresis, immunofixation, M-proteins, lytic lesions, etc." when you may simply be trying to address the question of what does this mean for me? Where do I go from here? Is there a possibility of cure? Patients and their families often take to the Internet where the information obtained can be overwhelming, overly technical, and difficult to negotiate to get to the answers they are looking for.

We try to help you through those difficulties. We start by defining myeloma and related conditions in lay terms. We explain the tests commonly used to diagnose and measure myeloma and then discuss the available treatments, which type of treatment options are appropriate for which type of patient, as well as the likely sequence in which these treatments will be used. We discuss the role of stem cell transplants and newer therapies in the treatment of myeloma as well as the social, financial, and insurance-related issues a patient may face and how best to deal with those non-medical issues that seem so often to get in the way. The Appendix also includes information regarding other resources that may help you in dealing with myeloma. We dedicate this book to the many thousands of patients who have fought this disease and those are presently fighting this disease and its effects.

PART ONE

The Basics

What is myeloma?

What is monoclonal gammopathy of undetermined significance (MGUS)?

What is a solitary plasmacytoma?

More ...

1. What is myeloma?

Myeloma (also known as **multiple myeloma**) is a cancer of the plasma cells that normally arises in the bone marrow but can also in rare instances arise at other sites. It usually results in the following:

- *Loss of normal marrow function* (blood cell production), leading to anemia and, less commonly, a shortage of normal white cells and platelets (blood cells that assist in clotting).
- *Overproduction of a single type of antibody* by the cancer cells. An **antibody** (also known as an **immunoglobulin**) is normally a blood protein that the body makes in response to infection and is designed to fight the infection by binding to the specific invading microbe. The body's normal production of immunoglobulin is **polyclonal** (meaning that the immunoglobulins produced are of many types and specificities). However, immunoglobulin made by a myeloma is typically **monoclonal**, or of a single type and specificity. This overproduced immunoglobulin (otherwise known as an **M-protein** or paraprotein) is usually of no use to the body, unlike normal immunoglobulin, and can sometimes cause harmful effects in itself. In some cases the abnormal immunoglobulin cannot be detected in the blood but is detectable in the urine. Some cases of myeloma have many or all of the other features but have no detectable M-protein in the blood or urine (nonsecretory myeloma). As the level of M-protein is an important way to follow the disease activity, nonsecretory myeloma may be difficult to monitor (see Question 17).

Multiple myeloma

a cancer of plasma cells usually arising in the bone marrow. Its features may include bone destruction, increased risk of infections, and kidney failure.

Antibody

a protein that is normally produced by the body's immune system to help fight infections. Each antibody usually has a specific target that it binds to and helps to eliminate. Normally many different types (specificities) of antibodies are made, targeting different microbes. In myeloma, an excess of one or a few antibodies is produced. Also called immunoglobulin.

Immunoglobulin

see *antibody*.

Polyclonal

arising from the division of many different cells.

- *Weakening of the bone* around sites where the bone marrow is involved. This usually takes the form of **lytic lesions** (areas that appear as punched-out holes in the skeleton on x-rays) where local involvement by myeloma has caused thinning of the bone. However, some patients develop generalized diffuse thinning of the bone, which can appear similar to severe osteoporosis ("normal" thinning of the bone with aging and after menopause). This thinning of the bone can result in fractures, which result in bone pain and sometimes produce skeletal instability.
- *Other complications* of myeloma that can occur include high blood calcium resulting from skeleton breakdown, kidney failure, and reduced normal antibody production, resulting in susceptibility to bacterial infections.

Several other related disorders of plasma cells exist that have some similarities to, but also important differences from, myeloma. These are described in the answers to Questions 2 through 5.

JWH: The first time I ever heard of multiple myeloma was when I was diagnosed with it. It is not very common, as you'll see later in these questions and answers, and the information available is scary. If you're the one with myeloma, you'll have noticed symptoms: fatigue, bone pain, and other problems (also discussed later). While you'll now have a diagnosis that explains the symptoms, you'll be very confused about what it is and what myeloma means. That's what this book is for: to give you the information you need to understand what you're battling and to help you make informed decisions about your treatment.

Monoclonal

arising from a single clone of abnormal cells. A clone means a population of identical cells, usually arising from the division of a single cell.

M-protein

also known as "paraprotein," excess antibody of one type that is produced in individuals with myeloma.

Lytic lesions

areas of bone thinning caused by myeloma and visible on an x-ray.

The Basics

Many of these early questions are very technical because myeloma is a very technical disease, one that is diagnosed and monitored through precise testing and definitions, not usually through x-rays taken looking for tumors and the like, as you might find with other cancers.

2. What is monoclonal gammopathy of undetermined significance (MGUS)?

MGUS is a relatively common condition in older patients, affecting up to 2% of patients over the age of 50. It is often discovered by chance when routine blood or urine testing is performed or while investigating another condition. Like myeloma, MGUS is characterized by an abnormal overproduction of a monoclonal protein or M-protein (see Question 1), which is seen in the blood or urine. However, the levels of the M-protein are usually lower than those seen in myeloma, and the patient has no symptoms. Bone marrow examination usually shows less than 10% involvement by plasma cells. The other features described in Question 1 are not present. In a proportion of patients, MGUS can progress over time (usually several years) to myeloma. However, in perhaps the majority of patients with MGUS, true myeloma will never occur. The diagnosis of MGUS is initially made by excluding myeloma with appropriate tests. Patients with MGUS are usually monitored for progression to full-blown myeloma, but no therapy is usually warranted in its absence.

Plasmacytoma
a localized collection of abnormal (usually monoclonal) plasma cells.

3. What is a solitary plasmacytoma?

A collection of myeloma cells is called a **plasmacytoma**. A **solitary plasmacytoma** occurs when only a single, localized deposit of abnormal plasma cells is found. This can occur at a single site in bone or in a soft-tissue area such as the respiratory tract or gut. The plasmacytoma may be discovered by chance or because of symptoms caused by its location. An M-protein may be found in the blood or urine, as in myeloma, but the levels of this protein are usually lower than seen in myeloma. When a solitary plasmacytoma occurs outside the bone or bone marrow, it may be possible to cure the disease with surgery, radiation therapy, or both. However, the disease can progress over time to full-blown myeloma; this is more likely when the marrow or bone is the primary site.

4. What is Waldenstrom's disease, and why is it relevant?

Waldenstrom's disease is a chronic disorder with some similarities to myeloma. Specifically, the abnormal cells produce high quantities of an M-protein. However, the M-protein produced is of the IgM class (see Question 6), and the bone abnormalities often seen in myeloma are usually absent. As in myeloma, anemia and kidney damage can result, but unlike myeloma, enlargement of the lymph glands is common, and the abnormal protein causes an increase in blood viscosity that can result in headaches, confusion, sleepiness, and visual disturbances. Waldenstrom's disease is often classified as a low-grade lymphoma (tumor of the lymph tissue) rather than a plasma cell disorder. Plasmapheresis (replacement of blood plasma using a specialized machine) can sometimes be effective in this disease but is rarely used in myeloma.

JWH: You should understand Waldenstrom's disease because it can look very much like myeloma. In fact, when I was

Waldenstrom's disease

sometimes referred to as Waldenstrom's macroglobulinemia. A plasma cell cancer that can be distinguished from myeloma by the production of abnormal IgM protein in the blood, which can cause increased blood viscosity. Bone destruction is usually absent.

first hospitalized with kidney failure and multiple other problems, the diagnosis was Waldenstrom's disease. I was in the ICU for 17 days, had chemotherapy for Waldenstrom's disease, and even had plasmapheresis many times. It was probably unnecessary (although there is some discussion now that plasmapheresis may be of benefit to myeloma patients in certain circumstances). I recommend that you ensure in whatever way you can (even through a second opinion by a pathologist) that the diagnosis is correct to ensure that the chosen course of treatment is the right one. For example, in Waldenstrom's disease the chemotherapy of choice is often melphalan, which makes production of cells for a later autologous stem cell transplant for treating myeloma much more difficult.

5. What is primary amyloidosis?

Primary amyloidosis

a disorder related to myeloma, characterized by impaired function of many organs resulting from deposition of an abnormal protein (M-protein) in tissues.

Primary amyloidosis is a disorder related to myeloma. It can sometimes be a complication of full-blown myeloma, but more commonly, although an M-protein can be detected in blood or urine, most of the other features of myeloma, including bone lesions, are absent. It results when abnormal plasma cells produce a particular type of M-protein that tends to be deposited in tissues and organs, resulting in impairment of their function. The organs most commonly involved include the tongue, gut, muscles, heart, kidneys, liver, spleen, skin, and nerves.

Among the symptoms most commonly resulting from amyloidosis are fatigue, numbness of hands and feet, weak hand grip, weight loss, shortness of breath, swelling of the extremities, enlarged tongue, swallowing difficulties, diarrhea, irregular heart rhythm, skin changes, and joint pain. The diagnosis is usually made through a biopsy of subcutaneous fat or other involved organ. A bone marrow biopsy, analysis of blood and urine protein content, and echocardiogram are also usually performed. Other tests, such as nerve conduction studies, may be necessary depending upon the symptoms.

The treatment of amyloidosis depends upon the organs involved and the severity of the involvement. Although it has conventionally been treated like myeloma, standard therapies for myeloma produce only limited benefit. Recent clinical trials suggest that stem cell transplantation may be a promising therapy for this disease, but it remains to be fully investigated.

6. What is immunoglobulin?

Immunoglobulin (also known as antibody) is a blood protein that the body makes in response to infection and is designed to fight the infection by binding specifically to the invading microbe. Normally, immunoglobulin contains at least two protein components—a larger **heavy chain** and a smaller **light chain**, which bind together to form the complete immunoglobulin. There are five types of heavy chains, which result in five different classes of immunoglobulin: IgG, IgA, IgM, IgD, and IgE. These classes differ from one another in their physical properties and their distribution within the body. For example, IgG can pass through the placenta from mother to baby but IgM cannot; and IgA is normally found in the lining of body cavities. There are two types of light chains, called kappa (κ) and lambda (λ).

Heavy chain

part of the biochemical structure of the antibody molecule.

Light chain

part of the biochemical structure of the antibody molecule.

Both heavy chains and light chains contain a constant region, which remains the same across all immunoglobulins of the same class, and a variable region, which is different for each immunoglobulin. The variable region of the immunoglobulin ensures that each immunoglobulin molecule has a unique target (that is, it has specificity). Whereas the normal range of immunoglobulins in the body is extremely diverse, in myeloma and other monoclonal plasma cell disorders, large quantities of a single class and specificity of immunoglobulin (M-protein) are produced by the myeloma cells (see Question 1), and normal immunoglobulin production is often suppressed.

JWH: Although the discussion of immunoglobulin sounds complex, become familiar with the terms, because tracking IgG (usually) or IgA (less commonly) is often the primary tool for determining how your disease is progressing or your condition is improving. The amount of those proteins shows up in the total protein number on your blood tests but is broken out by specific types in more precise tests. You will monitor those test results for a good indication of how your treatment is going.

7. What is a plasma cell?

Plasma cell

the type of cell that makes antibodies. It is usually produced by maturation of B-lymphocytes and is found in the bone marrow.

A **plasma cell** is one type of cell that is often found in the bone marrow but is also occasionally seen in other organs. Plasma cells are produced by the maturation of some types of lymph cells (B-lymphocytes). The primary function of a normal plasma cell is to produce an immunoglobulin (see Question 6). Normally, many different types of plasma cells produce a diverse collection of immunoglobulins in the blood; in myeloma and other monoclonal plasma cell disorders, however, the progeny of a single cancerous plasma cell proliferate without normal constraints and produce large quantities of a single type of immunoglobulin, which can then be detected in the blood or urine.

8. What is bone marrow?

Bone marrow is located in the central cavity of most flat bones and some long bones. It contains a mixture of fat stores and cells. The cells in the bone marrow perform many functions. **Hematopoietic** cells, a type of stem cell (see Question 65) in the bone marrow, produce blood cells such as red blood cells, white blood cells, and platelets. Although blood cells are present in relatively constant numbers in the blood, they are undergoing constant breakdown and renewal. Hematopoietic stem cells divide to produce new blood cells. In addition, bone marrow contains stromal cells that feed and support the hematopoietic cells, cells of the immune system such as lymphocytes and plasma cells, and cells of the phagocytic system designed to ingest and remove debris. When there is a cancer involving the bone marrow, such as leukemia or myeloma, these normal functions of bone marrow are often suppressed, leading to symptoms such as bleeding or anemia.

9. How does myeloma affect my ability to fight infection?

As myeloma progresses, normal immunoglobulin production is often severely suppressed. This can be detected in a blood test as low levels of normal immunoglobulin (hypogammaglobulinemia). This suppression impairs the body's ability to fight bacterial organisms. Patients with hypogammaglobulinemia

Bone marrow
a semiliquid fatty substance contained in the cavities of bones. Blood cells are manufactured here.

Hematopoietic
having to do with the production of blood cells.

The Basics

often develop recurrent bacterial infections, such as pneumonia and septicemia. The levels of normal immunoglobulin often recover upon successful treatment of myeloma. In some cases, however, replacement doses of immunoglobulin may be required (see Question 87).

In addition, the skeletal complications of myeloma, such as bone pain and fractures, often lead to poor mobility and impaired respiratory capacity, which in turn predispose the patient to pneumonia.

Also, some of the therapies used for myeloma, such as corticosteroids and some chemotherapy drugs, can temporarily impair other parts of the immune system, such as T-lymphocytes, further predisposing myeloma patients to specific infections.

10. What causes myeloma?

The exact causes of myeloma and other plasma cell disorders are poorly understood. There is evidence to suggest that in many cases, myeloma cells may be detectable in the body for many years or even decades before symptoms develop. Some patients develop myeloma as a progression of MGUS or a solitary plasmacytoma (see Question 2). The risk of developing myeloma is related to age—the disease is very uncommon in people under the age of 40, and most cases occur between the ages of 50 and 70. It is also more common in African-Americans than in Caucasians and in men than in women. There appears to be a slight genetic predisposition in that first-degree relatives of myeloma patients are at a slightly greater risk than average of developing the disease (see Question 86). Those exposed to large quantities of radiation (such as survivors of nuclear explosions) are also at increased risk, as are those employed in certain occupations associated with chemical exposure, such as oil industry workers and farmers. However, most patients who develop myeloma have no clear risk or causative factors for developing the disease.

11. Can myeloma be transmitted from one person to another?

There is no persuasive evidence that myeloma is contagious or related to a transmissible infectious agent. Your friends and relatives have no known risk of catching myeloma through contact with you.

The Basics

PART TWO

Diagnosis and Staging

How is myeloma diagnosed?

What is serum protein electrophoresis (SPEP)?

What is serum protein immunofixation (SIFE)?

What do the various stages of myeloma mean?

More ...

12. How is myeloma diagnosed?

Myeloma is usually first suspected because of symptoms or abnormalities discovered during a routine checkup or during the workup of an unrelated condition. The physician will then order a series of tests designed to confirm the diagnosis and determine the severity of the condition. Specific criteria have been developed to distinguish full-blown myeloma from related plasma cell disorders (see Questions 1–5). One of the most commonly used systems divides the diagnostic criteria into major and minor categories. (These are listed in Table 1.)

Tests may be performed on myeloma patients to establish the diagnosis and determine what stage of the dis-

TABLE 1   Diagnosis of Myeloma: Major and Minor Criteria

Under this diagnostic system, the diagnosis of myeloma requires at least two major criteria or one major plus one minor criterion or three minor criteria. However, some physicians may use an alternative system of criteria to establish the diagnosis.

Major criteria

  i. Plasmacytoma (abnormal collection of plasma cells) is found on tissue biopsy
 ii. Plasma cells constitute $\geq$ 30% of bone marrow cells on a biopsy
iii. Monoclonal protein seen on an assessment of blood serum or urine is quantitated to be > 3 g/dl for IgG, > 2 g for IgA, or > 1 g/24 hours of immunoglobulin present in urine

Minor criteria

  i. Plasma cells make up 10–30% of bone marrow cells
 ii. Monoclonal protein is found but at lower levels than those described for the major criteria
iii. Lytic lesions (localized areas of bone thinning) are seen on bone x-rays
 iv. Low levels of normal immunoglobulin are found: IgM < 0.05 g/dl, IgA < 0.1 g/dl, IgG < 0.6 g/dl

ease the patient is in (see Question 22) as well as to provide other information relevant to the patient's prognosis and ability to tolerate therapy. Several tests are performed initially when myeloma is suspected and then at periodic intervals to reassess the status of the disease. Many of the tests performed on myeloma patients measure the level and assess the type of M-protein that is present in the blood (serum) and the urine. These include the SPEP, SIFE, QIG, UPEP, UIFE, and free-light-chain tests described in the answers to Questions 13 through 18.

13. What is serum protein electrophoresis (SPEP)?

In an **SPEP** test, the technician first removes red blood cells and clotting proteins from the drawn blood. The resulting serum is then placed on an agar gel, and an electrical current is applied. The procedure separates serum proteins into separate groups based upon their size and charge. This test allows the identification of an abnormal monoclonal band of immunoglobulin, which is called a paraprotein, M-protein, M-spike, or M-component. The electrophoresis also enables an approximate quantitation of the M-protein, which can be used to follow the disease's response to therapy.

SPEP (serum protein electrophoresis)
a biochemical technique that separates and visualizes different proteins found in blood serum by running them on a gel under an electric current.

JWH: The M-protein is often used as a major indicator of the status of your myeloma. It can be monitored very closely and as often as needed. The effectiveness of various treatments is usually reflected directly in the M-protein number.

14. What is serum protein immunofixation (SIFE)?

The **SIFE** test is used to identify the exact subtype of monoclonal immunoglobulin present (see Question 6), indicating whether it is an IgG, IgA, or IgD and whether its light chain is a kappa or lambda chain. This test can also detect free light chains. The proportion of patients with each different type of myeloma is approximately as follows:

IgG: 55%

IgA: 25%

Light chain only: 15%

Nonsecretory: 2%

IgD: 1–2%

IgM, IgE, or biclonal: rare

The SIFE test is more sensitive than the SPEP test and is therefore used to monitor patients with very low levels of M-protein. A negative SIFE test in serum and urine is normally necessary to obtain a complete response to therapy in myeloma.

15. What is the quantitative immunoglobulins (QIG) measurement?

The **QIG** test measures the levels of specific subtypes of immunoglobulin in the serum—such as IgG, IgA, and IgM (see Question 6)—and provides relatively accurate quantification, expressed as g/dl or mg/dl. The measurements do not distinguish between normal (polyclonal) and abnormal (monoclonal) immunoglobulin, and the value obtained is usually a composite of the two. This test is particularly useful when the levels of the M-protein are very high, leading to very elevated levels of the immunoglobulin in question. In such cases, the fall in the level of the quantitatively measured immunoglobulin can be used to determine how good the response obtained to a therapy is. This test is therefore most often performed repeatedly to assess disease status. The QIG analysis can also be used to determine the degree to which the levels of other immunoglobulins, besides the category to which the M-component belongs, are being suppressed. For example, it can be used to measure a reduction of IgA levels in a patient with IgG myeloma.

16. How are immunoglobulins assessed in the urine?

Urine protein electrophoresis (UPEP) and urine immunofixation (UIFE) are performed on urine like the similar tests performed on serum. Traditionally, excretion of excess free immunoglobulin light chains in the urine was assessed by the Bence-Jones test—involving precipitating proteins through heating and then redissolving them through boiling. UIFE and UPEP are more commonly performed now. However, free-light-chain excretion in myeloma patients is still referred to as Bence-Jones proteinuria.

Urine immunoglobulin excretion is measured by collecting a 24-hour specimen of urine and measuring the total immunoglobulin excretion during that period. In patients who have a detectable light-chain immunoglobulin only in the urine, with little or no serum M-protein, a series of tests of 24-hour urine immunoglobulin excretion be the primary way of determining how the disease has responded to therapy.

17. What is the Freelite test?

The **Freelite test** is a recently developed test that measures free light chains (see Question 6) in the serum or the urine. It is a more accurate method of measuring the M-protein in patients with light-chain myeloma. It may also detect and measure an otherwise undetectable light chain in patients previously thought to have nonsecretory myeloma (one in which no M-protein is made). This test makes identifying the myeloma and measuring the response to therapy much easier in those cases. If you are told you have a nonsecretory myeloma or a light-chain-only myeloma, the Freelite test may be of benefit in your case.

18. What is a bone marrow biopsy?

During a **bone marrow biopsy**, the physician obtains a small amount of the fluid within the bone marrow cavity (aspirate), with or without a small piece of bone (biopsy) to examine under the microscope. The procedure is usually performed under local anesthetic from the back of one of the large hip bones (posterior iliac crest). To allow access to the posterior iliac crest, the patient is placed either on his or her side in a fetal position or flat on his or her stomach (the position chosen usually depends upon the physician's preference and the patient's comfort—a good sample of marrow is easily obtained using either position). Occasionally, alternative sites on the body have to be used, such as the front bones of the pelvis (anterior iliac crest) or the breast bone (sternum).

When performed by an experienced physician, the procedure takes 20 to 30 minutes or less. The patient may experience some pain or discomfort when the local anesthetic is being inserted. When the marrow is aspirated, there may be a very temporary painful sensation that to some people feels like a jolt of electricity. This sensation usually lasts only while the physician is applying suction to aspirate the marrow fluid (typically 1 second or so). If the patient is warned, he or she can usually tolerate this sensation without difficulty. General anesthetic and oral or intravenous painkillers are usually not necessary. If patients are particulary anxious, this may be relieved by using anti-anxiety medication prior to the procedure, such as Ativan. Once the procedure is completed, there should be no residual pain—some patients feel a little discomfort in the region that lasts for a day or so.

The bone marrow aspirate/biopsy enables the physician to determine what percentage of the bone marrow cells are plasma cells (normally < 5%). This percentage is important to know in diagnosing and subsequently monitoring myeloma and in determining the disease's response to therapy. It is important to understand that marrow involvement by myeloma can be patchy, and therefore the percentage of plasma cells can vary somewhat from biopsy to biopsy without there being a true change in the degree of involvement.

JWH: The bone marrow biopsy or aspiration is a common procedure in the treatment of myeloma. It allows the physician to actually see the plasma cells in the bone marrow, which is very helpful for treatment and diagnosis. But I must say that it is also probably thought by most myeloma patients to be the most unpleasant of the normal procedures encountered, more so even than chemotherapy. It doesn't

Diagnosis and Staging

take very long, but it is sharply painful for that brief time. They can numb the skin and muscle right down to the bone, but not inside the bone. I don't want to alarm you if you're about to endure one of these procedures, but you should be aware of it. It will be over quickly, and the soreness lasts only a couple of days. Some patients are unenthusiastic about walking right after a biopsy, while others are not as bothered by it. I was usually able to run the next morning (as I've tried to do throughout my treatment, subject to my bones strengthening enough to get the green light from my doctor).

19. What special tests can be performed on the bone marrow biopsy specimen?

Other tests that can be performed upon the myeloma cells in the bone marrow aspirate are as follows: **Flow cytometry** looks at which proteins the myeloma cells have on their surface. This may allow a more precise determination of their number and sometimes helps distinguish abnormal from normal plasma cells. **Cytogenetics** looks at the chromosomes within the myeloma plasma cells. This can be done one of two ways. The first involves inducing obtained myeloma cells to divide and then examining the chromosomes under the microscope during cell division. Alternatively, a specialized technique called fluorescence in-situ hybridization, or FISH, examines chromosomes even in nondividing cells, using fluorescent probes. Abnormalities of chromosome 13 in particular have been shown to have prognostic value in myeloma.

In some centers, a **plasma cell labeling index (PCLI)** is performed. This is a measure of the rate of proliferation of the myeloma cells and has been shown to have some prognostic value. However, it is laborious to per-

Flow cytometry

a test performed on blood or bone marrow that detects the amount and types of proteins that are present on or in cells.

Cytogenetic analysis

a technique used to visualize chromosomes in cells and thus detect whether abnormalities are present.

Plasma cell labeling index (PCLI)

a test used to measure the rate of growth of myeloma cells.

form, and the prognostic information from a PCLI can be obtained using other tests.

20. How is the skeleton evaluated for bone abnormalities caused by myeloma?

The skeleton is most commonly assessed using a an *x-ray skeletal survey*. X-rays are taken of all the bones in the body, and these are evaluated for areas of bone thinning (lytic lesions), generalized osteoporosis, and fractures (including spinal compression fractures). **Magnetic resonance imaging (MRI)** of the spine is sometimes also performed. This can identify lytic lesions that are not visible on plain x-rays and is also useful if it is suspected that the patient's myeloma is causing spinal cord compression.

21. What other routine blood tests are performed to assess myeloma?

The physician will also perform a routine **complete blood count (CBC)** to assess whether there is anemia or any other abnormality of blood cells, and a **chemistry profile** to identify kidney dysfunction or high blood calcium caused by the myeloma. The **beta-2-microglobulin level (B2M)** is an important prognostic factor in myeloma. The level of B2M reflects the amount of myeloma present. It should be performed as part of the initial assessment and is also used to follow the patient's disease in some cases. However, it can be falsely elevated in the presence of kidney failure. **Lactate dehydrogenase (LDH)** is an enzyme protein present inside cells. High levels of LDH in the blood have been shown to indicate a worse prognosis in myeloma.

JWH: As your treatment progresses, these blood tests will become even more important, as much of the therapy has

X-ray skeletal survey

A procedure in which x-rays of all the bones in the body are taken to identify bone abnormalities caused by myeloma.

Magnetic resonance imaging (MRI)

a type of imaging of the inside of the body that relies on placing the patient in a strong magnetic field and detecting the changes caused in the tissues by that magnetic field.

Complete blood count (CBC)

a laboratory test that measures the number of red cells, white cells, and platelet cells in the blood and also measures the concentration of hemoglobin.

Chemistry profile

a test that measures the levels of various chemicals in the blood.

Beta-2-micro-globulin level (B2M)

a protein whose levels in blood indicate how much myeloma is present in the body. Its level is an indicator of prognosis.

Diagnosis and Staging

*implications for other parts of your body—such as the
ability to produce red blood cells; the ability to fight
infection, as shown by the white blood cell level; and the
ability to clot in case of bleeding, as shown by the
platelet level.*

22. What do the various stages of myeloma mean?

In most cancers, the disease **stage** reflects the extent of
spread of the tumor and the prognosis of the patient.
Myeloma is not typically localized to one site when it
is diagnosed. Usually the bone marrow is widely infil-
trated by the abnormal plasma cells. In myeloma, the
stage reflects the size of the myeloma burden (the
number of myeloma cells in the body) and the prognosis of the patient. The most commonly used staging
system for myeloma is that developed by Durie and
Salmon (Durie-Salmon staging system). In this system, three stages are defined as follows:

Stage I: A relatively small number of myeloma cells are
present throughout the body, There may be no symptoms arising from the disease. The number of red
blood cells and the amount of calcium in the blood are
normal or almost normal. The amount of M-protein
in the blood or urine is low.

Stage II: A moderate number of myeloma cells are
present in the body (the myeloma falls between the
criteria for Stages I and III).

Stage III: A large number of myeloma cells are present throughout the body. One or more of the following is present:

• Anemia, a decrease in the level of hemoglobin in
the blood

- High levels of calcium in the blood, because the bones are being damaged
- More than three areas of lytic bone lesions
- High levels of M-protein in the blood or urine

Stages I through III are further subclassified according to whether renal failure is absent (A) or present (B).

Details regarding the Durie-Salmon staging system are provided in Table 2.

JWH: Staging is important, but don't assume that the stage you're in at diagnosis determines how it is all going to go. If, for example, you're Stage IIIB when diagnosed—as I was—don't assume that all is lost. Treatment options have improved dramatically over the last few years, and you need to be ready to fight.

23. What are smoldering myeloma and indolent myeloma?

These are two conditions that can be distinguished from active multiple myeloma because they often do not require any therapy initially. It is currently felt that there is not much distinction between these two types of myeloma and that they should be regarded as essentially the same entity.

Smoldering multiple myeloma (SMM): Patients with SMM satisfy the diagnostic criteria for multiple myeloma (see Question 12 and Table 1) and can therefore be distinguished from patients with MGUS. However, they have no symptoms and are not affected by the anemia, bone disease, renal failure, and frequent infections that characterize active multiple myeloma. In patients with SMM, the myeloma may be static and may not progress for months or years. Thus, these patients are observed and are usually treated only if

Smoldering multiple myeloma (SMM)

a condition in which the criteria for a diagnosis of myeloma are met but the patient is in an early stage of the disease, with no symptoms.

TABLE 2   The Durie-Salmon Staging System

Stage	Criteria	Estimated myeloma cell mass
I	All of the following: • Hemoglobin value < 10 g/dl • Serum calcium value normal or ≥ 12 mg/dl • Absence of anemia, renal failure, hypercalcemia, and lytic bone lesions • Low M-component production rate • IgG value < 5 g/dl; IgA value < 3 g/dl • Bence-Jones protein < 4 g/24 h	< 0.6 cells × 10^{12}/m² (low cell mass)
II	Fitting neither Stage I nor Stage III	0.6–1.2 cells × 10^{12}/m² (intermediate cell mass)
III	One or more of the following: • Hemoglobin value < 8.5 g/dl • Serum calcium value > 12 mg/dl • Advanced lytic bone lesions (scale 3) • High M-component production rate • IgG value > 7 g/dl; IgA value > 5 g/dl • Bence-Jones protein > 12 g/24 h	> 1.2 cells × 10^{12}/m² (high cell mass)

Subclassification (either A or B)

A: Relatively normal renal function (serum creatinine value < 2.0 mg/dl)

B: Abnormal renal function (serum creatinine value ≥ 2.0 mg/dl)

Indolent multiple myeloma (IMM)

similar to SMM, though patients with IMM may have mild anemia or a few bone lesions.

their disease progresses. About 5% of myeloma patients are classified with SMM at diagnosis.

Indolent multiple myeloma (IMM): Patients with IMM also have no symptoms. They have a monoclonal protein and an increased number of plasma cells in the bone marrow, as in SMM. However, unlike patients with SMM, they may also have mild anemia or a few bone lesions. Patients with indolent myeloma are typically monitored every 3 months and are treated if the disease begins to progress.

For details regarding SMM and IMM, see Table 3.

24. What are the symptoms of myeloma?

Myeloma can cause bone pain, either directly through lytic lesions (essentially, thinning or holes in the bones) or through fractures caused by weakening of the bone by the myeloma lesions. When the fractures occur following little or no trauma, they are called **pathological fractures**. Bone pain from myeloma often affects multiple sites and can be very severe, requiring strong pain medication to control. Fractures in the spine can cause compression of the vertebral bodies (bones of the spine), which can cause loss of height in addition to bone pain. Bone pain and fractures can result in limitation of mobility, which can severely impair quality of life and predispose the patient to other complications such as pneumonia and blood clots in the legs. Sometimes fractures within the spine and/or deposits of myeloma within the spinal canal can cause **spinal cord compression**. This often starts off with back pain, which can shoot down the legs and can be accompanied by numbness of the legs and buttocks. This is a medical emergency because if left untreated it can rapidly cause paralysis of the legs and loss of bladder and bowel control.

Some symptoms of myeloma may be related to abnormalities in the blood caused by the disease. Anemia is a common problem in advanced myeloma and can

Diagnosis and Staging

Pathological fracture

a fracture that occurs in a bone that is weakened by a disease process. The fracture typically occurs following no trauma or minimal trauma that would be insufficient to cause a fracture in a normal bone.

Spinal cord compression

compression of the spinal cord (usually by a tumor or a spinal fracture), resulting in neurological symptoms. This is a medical emergency requiring rapid intervention to prevent long-term paralysis.

TABLE 3 Classification of Patients with Multiple Myeloma and MGUS

Type	Features	Management
Monoclonal gammopathy of undetermined significance (MGUS)	• Serum M-protein < 3 g/dl (IgG); < 2g/dl(IgA) • Bone marrow plasma cells < 10% if done • Absence of anemia, renal failure, hypercalcemia, and lytic bone lesions	Observation, with treatment when disease progresses
Smoldering multiple myeloma (SMM)	• Serum M-protein > 3 g/dl (IgG); > 2g/dl (IgA) *and* • Bone marrow plasma cells < 10% if done • Absence of anemia, renal failure, hypercalcemia, and lytic bone lesions	Observation, with treatment when disease progresses
Indolent multiple myeloma (IMM)	• Presence of serum/urine M-protein • Bone marrow plasmacytosis • Mild anemia or few small lytic bone lesions • Absence of symptoms	Monitoring every 3 months, with treatment beginning at disease progression
Symptomatic multiple myeloma	• Presence of serum/urine M-protein • Bone marrow plasmacytosis • Anemia, renal failure, hypercalcemia, or lytic bone lesions • Patients with primary systematic amyloidosis and bone marrow plasma cells $\geq$ 30% are considered to have both MM and amyloidosis	Treat

manifest as increased fatigue, shortness of breath on exertion, dizziness, and palpitations. Significantly, though, it may be the first indication of myeloma. Increased blood calcium can accompany lytic bone lesions. It can manifest as nausea, confusion, constipation, increased amounts of urine, and thirst. Renal failure is a feature of some types of myeloma; it can cause drowsiness, confusion, and heavy breathing.

A reduction in normal immunoglobulin levels is common in advanced myeloma. It can result in increased risk of bacterial infections, particularly bronchitis and pneumonias.

Occasionally, myeloma can result in multiple masses (cancerous lumps) involving not just the bone but other organ systems. Often such "soft-tissue" masses arise originally in bone but spread out to adjacent skin, muscle, fat, and so on. This is usually a sign of more aggressive and rapidly advancing disease (see Question 26).

Like all cancers, advanced myeloma can result in loss of appetite and weight loss, which can lead to further weakening of muscles already affected by bone fractures and immobility. It is important that malnutrition resulting from advanced myeloma be recognized, as it can respond to nutritional supplements, appetite stimulants, and direct treatment of the myeloma.

Rarely, the abnormal immunoglobulin made by the myeloma may target some normal protein in the body. If that happens, tissues bearing that protein may be damaged by the immunoglobulin. For example, an abnormal immunoglobulin that targets nerve cells can cause numbness and pain of the arms and legs (peripheral neuropathy), although this symptom is much more commonly a side effect of the treatments used for myeloma.

Amyloidosis can occur as a complication in some cases of myeloma. This results when the myeloma protein produces insoluble deposits in vital organs, impairing their function. Symptoms of amyloidosis are described in Question 5.

25. Does myeloma spread like other cancers?

Myeloma can sometimes occur as a localized disease known as solitary plasmacytoma (see Question 3). However, usually the myeloma cells are widely spread throughout the bone marrow at diagnosis. The bone marrow involvement can be patchy—sometimes with wide discrepancies between marrow biopsies performed at different sites on the body. In most cases of myeloma, the abnormal plasma cells remain within the bone marrow, causing failure of normal marrow function and areas of adjacent bone thinning (lytic lesions). Sometimes the myeloma cells can extend from the bone marrow or bone into surrounding soft tissues. When this occurs in the spinal canal, it can cause spinal cord compression. Thus, although in the majority of cases myeloma does not spread widely to multiple organs of the body like other malignant tumors, there are exceptions. Rarely, myeloma cells can spill extensively into the blood. When this happens, the disease is called plasma cell leukemia and has a worse prognosis.

26. What is plasmablastic myeloma?

In rare cases, the myeloma cells are more immature in their appearance than typical plasma cells. These cells look like plasmablasts (precursors of plasma cells). Cases of **plasmablastic myeloma** are often associated with an elevated blood LDH (see Question 21). This form of the disease is usually more aggressive than typical myeloma and has a worse prognosis. It may involve sites such as muscle, skin, and vital organs that are not normally invaded by myeloma. Plasmablastic

Plasmablastic myeloma

an aggressive type of myeloma characterized by rapid growth of the abnormal cells and an elevated LDH level.

myeloma may require alternative treatments such as those used in aggressive lymph cancers.

27. What determines the prognosis in myeloma?

The prognosis of patients with myeloma is highly variable—survival can be less than 1 year from diagnosis in some patients and more than 10 years from diagnosis in others. Several factors can be assessed at diagnosis that have been shown to correlate with prognosis in patients with myeloma. Among the factors that have been shown to be important in this regard are the following:

Durie-Salmon stage

Age at diagnosis

Beta-2 microglobulin level (blood)

LDH level (blood)

Plasma cell labeling index

C-reactive protein level (blood)

Albumin level (blood)

Type and level of M-protein (blood or urine)

Presence of chromosome 13 abnormalities on cyto-genetic or FISH testing (bone marrow)

Presence of kidney failure

Presence of increased blood calcium

Plasmablastic appearance to myeloma cells (bone marrow)

See Questions 13–21 for further information on these tests.

Your physician may use a selection of these factors to help determine your prognosis at diagnosis. The exact tests used will vary based upon your physician's preference and what is available locally. Sometimes groups of these prognostic factors can be put together to provide approximate average survival times for patients with a specific combination of factors. For example, patients with normal cytogenetics and a B2M of less than 2.5 mg/L have a survival of more than 111 months on average. In contrast, patients with abnormalities of chromosome 13 and a B2M of greater than 2.5 mg/L have a survival of 22 months on average.

It is important to appreciate that the values quoted by such systems are an *average*, meaning that some patients will live longer and some less than the stated value. Individual patients with exactly the same prognosis may have quite different outcomes based upon chance and individual variations that the prognostic factor system may not have taken into account. Furthermore, as therapeutic advances occur, survival predicted based upon past statistics may not remain accurate. Thus, methods for determining prognosis are simply a guide to how the myeloma might behave in an individual patient, and they are best used to identify patients who may require more (or less) aggressive therapy rather than to accurately predict the survival of an individual patient.

JWH: As a patient, you really want to know the answer to this question right away. It's the typical question you might see in a movie: "How long do I have, doc?" But the answer isn't simple. Don't place too much reliance on data or statistics to tell you how your own treatment will come out. As another cancer patient said to me once, "You're not a statistic. This disease has never encountered you before."

A lot of data is available regarding survival statistics in myeloma, and generally it isn't good. But keep a few things in mind. Myeloma has been around (identified) since the late 19th century. Survival back then was short. As treatment has progressed, survival rates have gotten much better. Most significantly, though, treatments in the last decade have probably made more progress than in the 50 years before that put together. Numerous teaching hospitals are now dedicating much more effort to studying myeloma, and they are making progress. Several organizations have been founded that are dedicated to researching myeloma, which has not received as much attention as other cancers in the past due to the lower numbers of patients. (Approximately 15,000 new cases of myeloma are diagnosed in the United States each year, compared to over 200,000 cases of lung cancer.)

Additionally, treatments are now being used that could provide long-term relief, and these treatments don't figure into the data. It is much better to be diagnosed with myeloma today than it was 10 or 20 years ago. And with each year of survival, the odds of a truly beneficial long-term course of treatment increase.

28. How should I cope with the diagnosis of myeloma?

The diagnosis of myeloma, like that of any life-threatening illness, can produce powerful emotions in both you the patient and your loved ones. The emotions felt can include shock, denial, anger, fear, helplessness, and grief. These emotions can be felt simultaneously or in sequence and are a normal part of coming to terms with the diagnosis. At this time, the support and understanding of other individuals

Diagnosis and Staging

can be invaluable. Patients can turn to various combinations of family, friends, neighbors, religious and social support groups, and other myeloma survivors for this assistance. Generally, an open discussion of your diagnosis, its implications, and your emotions and needs with others is most productive in this situation. The use of medications to relieve anxiety, help you sleep, and elevate your mood can be extremely useful in allowing you to cope with your diagnosis, and you should not feel ashamed to discuss your psychological needs with your physician and caregivers. Some techniques that do not rely upon medication, such as meditation and relaxation techniques, can also be useful for some patients. Although you may not have thought much about emotional health before, it is important to use the techniques available to optimize your emotional status so that you are able to undergo treatment and have the determination you'll need to overcome the challenges posed by your disease.

JWH: I have to say that I was really knocked down when I was diagnosed. I was 48 years old and had five children (still do). I was struck with a deep sense of sadness and loss, and I began to lose heart about the future. I went from skiing with my family at Lake Tahoe to being in the intensive care unit in three days. I had complete kidney failure and 100% cancerous bone marrow. I was getting those looks from doctors that you hope never to see. But I was surrounded by friends and family who encouraged me. Who walked with me every day when I got out of the hospital to build my strength back up. Who read to me and laughed with me. My wife helped sustain me by being my unfailing companion. Reach out to those people in your life who can help you. Lean on them. Don't be too proud. You'll find warmth and kindness you didn't know existed from people you wouldn't expect it from.

I am a Christian, and I found tremendous comfort in thinking of things from an eternal perspective. If you are a person of faith, seek out the depth of your faith to support you through this time. If you are not, think of what gives you the deepest comfort and assurance. We all should think broadly and of others. Think of how you can reach out to others, especially other patients, to help them, which will in turn help you.

29. Should I seek a second opinion?

A second opinion is not always necessary but can be useful for some patients. It allows you to hear about your diagnosis and treatment plan from a second oncologist. Having the same issues explained by two different physicians in their different styles may allow you to comprehend the ideas presented more completely. It can also be reassuring to find out that a second oncologist agrees with the diagnosis and treatment plan suggested by your primary oncologist. If you have any doubts about the statements of your primary oncologist or the compatibility of his or her style and approach with your preferences, a second opinion may allow you to sample an alternative physician to whom you may later elect to transfer your care. If you are interested in finding out about clinical trials of newer therapies for your myeloma, a second opinion may also make you aware of alternative trials that may be preferable to you.

There are some potential disadvantages to seeking a second opinion. Some patients may find differences of opinion between the two physicians to be distressing and emotionally draining. It is important to recognize that there are often many different ways to correctly diagnose and treat a cancer. Thus, some of the differences uncovered through a second opinion may simply reflect valid differences in opinion and approach between two physicians who are equally informed and competent. Only occasionally does a difference in opinion reveal substandard care by one physician. However, some patients find the uncertainty highlighted by even these valid differences to be disconcerting. Also, a second opinion may consume valuable time and produce a delay in therapy. Sometimes, if clearly conflicting opinions are obtained from the two physicians, a third opinion is necessary to resolve the differences.

For most patients, a second opinion is a useful exercise. However, some patients obtain multiple opinions from many different physicians and institutions. This can be counterproductive, causing indecision and delays, and should be avoided.

Some patients feel uncomfortable about obtaining a second opinion because they feel it will cause offense to their primary oncologist. However, it is your right to obtain such an opinion, and most oncologists understand that it is a useful exercise in your attempts to better understand the disease you are facing and the therapies offered to you.

JWH: I went through the issue of whether to get a second opinion twice. The first time was after I was released from the hospital, to ensure that my diagnosis (Waldenstrom's disease) was correct. It wasn't. If I hadn't gotten a second opinion, I think it is likely my treatment would have gone dramatically off course, and I am not confident I would be where I am today (working full time as an attorney, writing novels, running every day, traveling to Europe, and raising a family). So my first "second opinion" was critical to my care. I believe the necessity of that diagnostic second opinion is inversely related to the experience your oncologist has had in blood cancers. If that person has a lot of experience with Waldenstrom's disease, and myeloma, you may be okay. But what's the harm in being sure, when the treatment for one may preclude the correct treatment for the other?

The second "second opinion" I got was related to what the best treatment was for myeloma. One nationally known doctor recommended drug therapy only and not a bone marrow transplant; the other recommended the transplant. Again, I thought it was good for me to hear both of those approaches advocated, so I could decide between them. (More about that actual decision later.)

In summary, if you think a second opinion might be of benefit, you should do it. And many insurance companies will pay for it.

30. How do I arrange for a second opinion?

It is best to arrange for a second opinion before you begin your therapy. You should discuss the urgency of the planned therapy with your primary oncologist first. Most oncology treatments are not emergency procedures, and there is time (a period of days to weeks and sometimes longer, depending on your specific case) during which a second opinion can be sought. However, your primary oncologist will identify any reasons for beginning therapy immediately if such an emergency exists. Sometimes you may need a second opinion after therapy is begun. Usually this need arises when a change of therapy is planned—for example, if your current therapy is no longer working and you are being offered a different therapy.

It is best to obtain a second opinion from a physician who is truly independent of your primary oncologist. This usually means seeing a doctor who works at a different institution from your primary oncologist. Second opinions are recognized as part of your treatment plan and are therefore paid for by most insurance companies. However, in some cases your insurance may deny such a visit and you may have to pay for the opinion out of your own pocket.

It can often be helpful to seek the opinion of a physician who specializes in myeloma or bone marrow–related cancer rather than a general oncologist. Such specialists are usually found in university teaching hospitals or other large cancer centers (such as cancer centers designated by the National Cancer Institute [www.cancer.gov]). It is usually possible to call the "new patient office" of such a center and request the oncologist or hematologist who specializes in myeloma. Such physicians generally see many more myeloma cases than a regular oncologist and may be more aware of the latest developments in this field. However, seeing such a specialist does not mean that you should necessarily transfer your care to him or her. Many patients value the local availability and personal touch of their primary oncologist. Obtaining a second opinion from the specialist can allow you to take advantage of the special skills of both physicians.

In order to obtain your opinion, it is usually necessary to gather copies of your medical records, x-rays and scans, and pathology slides of any biopsies used to make the diagnosis. The pathologists at the institution where you are seeking the second opinion will usually perform their own second opinion on your pathology slides.

JWH: I also recommend that you get a second opinion from an expert in the field. Most local oncologists simply won't have treated many myeloma patients. You should talk to someone who has. In addition to checking out web sites, find myeloma patients who have already been through this process and ask them for recommendations. There are e-mail lists of people who have myeloma or are caregivers to others who do. They can be a wonderful source of information on good doctors to see for a second opinion. You might want to join the e-mail list sponsored by the Association of Cancer Online Resources (see Question 95), where such information is exchanged regularly. I also endorse getting a second opinion on the pathology findings that diagnosed your multiple myeloma. It pays to be sure. As I've said, my initial diagnosis was wrong, and that was after a pathology report. I then had the slides read by three other pathologists, who came to the correct conclusion.

PART THREE

Treatment Options

Should all cases of myeloma receive treatment?

What options are available for the treatment of myeloma?

What is the usual sequence of treatments for myeloma?

More . . .

31. Should all cases of myeloma receive treatment?

Patients in a very early stage of the disease may not immediately require treatment directed against the myeloma cells. This is often the case if the myeloma is not causing any symptoms (for example, in smoldering myeloma or indolent myeloma—see Question 23). MGUS (see Question 2) almost never requires specific therapy because there are no symptoms to treat, and the treatment has not been shown to delay or avoid progression to a more advanced (or symptomatic) stage. However, if there are symptoms that can be attributed to the myeloma (see Question 24), if the disease is in an advanced stage, or if the myeloma has caused damage to the skeleton such that fractures are imminent, therapy directed against the myeloma cells is used. Patients who are very elderly or who have many unrelated medical conditions that are debilitating are sometimes not offered aggressive antimyeloma therapy, as these patients are at increased risk of side effects from the therapy itself.

32. What options are available for the treatment of myeloma?

Four major types of treatment are used to treat patients with myeloma:

- *Drug therapy* involves the use of a drug (usually either intravenous or oral) to attack the myeloma cells. The drug used can be either a **chemotherapy** drug (a drug that targets all rapidly dividing cells) or other agents including novel targeted therapies.

- *Radiation therapy* uses x-rays or other forms of high-energy rays aimed at areas of the body involved by the myeloma to kill the myeloma cells and relieve symptoms. This approach usually does not treat the whole body (as drug therapy does) and is therefore used to treat symptomatic involvement of a localized area of the body by myeloma (such as the spine).
- *Immunotherapy* stimulates the body's immune system to fight the myeloma. The most commonly used form of immunotherapy is allogeneic bone marrow or stem cell transplantation (see Questions 65–78). However, vaccine-based approaches and other forms of experimental immune therapies are also being studied as part of clinical trials.
- *Ancillary therapies* do not directly target the myeloma cells but instead treat, relieve, or prevent some complication of myeloma. The most commonly used ancillary therapies are bisphosphonates (Aredia and Zometa) to protect the skeleton and treat increased blood calcium, intravenous immunoglobulin (IVIG) to treat low blood levels of normal antibodies, and vertebroplasty/kyphoplasty (a surgical technique that relieves pain caused by collapse fractures of the spinal bones).

Radiation therapy
treatment of cancer using x-rays or electron beam therapy.

Immunotherapy
a type of treatment that uses the body's immune system to fight disease.

Ancillary therapies
medical treatments used to prevent or relieve complications of a disease, rather than the disease itself.

Treatment Options

33. What is the usual sequence of treatments for myeloma?

The initial objective of treatment for myeloma is to relieve symptoms and prevent complications of the disease by decreasing the number of myeloma cells that are

Induction therapy
initial phase of treat-
ment, which
attempts to decrease
the number of dis-
ease cells in order to
relieve symptoms
and prevent compli-
cations.

Remission
regression of the
patient's disease,
with an accompany-
ing improvement in
symptoms.

present in the body. This initial phase of the treatment is sometimes called **induction therapy** or **remission induction**. Usually a combination of chemotherapy and corticosteroids (either dexamethasone or prednisone) is used for this purpose. However, some physicians use thalidomide and dexamethasone (TD) or pulse dexamethasone alone (D), or even BLT (Biaxin, low-dose thalidomide) or BLT-D (BLT with dexamethasone) as alternative types of induction therapy. You should discuss the pros and cons of the different induction therapy regimens carefully with your oncologist.

In general, the use of a regimen such as VAD (vincristine, Adriamycin, and dexamethasone) or TD is preferred in patients who have the prospect of going on to stem cell transplant therapy (see Questions 65–78). These regimens appear to have two main advantages over an older regimen called melphalan and prednisone (M&P): (1) It seems to minimize impairment of the stem cells, so that they can later be collected for autologous transplantation; and (2) the response is usually achieved more quickly. However, the overall number of patients who eventually achieve a response seems to be about the same with either regimen. The VAD regimen requires intravenous therapy (usually by continuous infusion for 4 days each month). Some other regimens, such as M&P, TD, or dexamethasone alone, are completely oral. Usually, 3 to 6 cycles of one of these induction therapy regimens is administered (each cycle typically lasts a month).

Patients are usually also begun upon bisphosphonate therapy (Aredia or Zometa) at diagnosis. This is an ancillary therapy administered once a month and has been shown to delay or prevent weakening of the skeleton by the myeloma. It is usually continued for at least 2 years and may be continued indefinitely.

Patients who show evidence of a response to induction therapy usually proceed to high-dose chemotherapy and autologous stem cell support (HDC-ASCS) (see Question 68). Although some controversy still exists, there is evidence that most myeloma patients benefit from at least one cycle of HDC-ASCS, and some patients may benefit from two such cycles. Once the HDC-ASCS has been administered, the patient is often followed without therapy until the disease shows laboratory evidence of recurrence or relapse. As the remission period following HDC-ASCS can range from several months to several years, this allows patients to enjoy time without active therapy and its associated side effects. Some physicians administer "maintenance" therapy during this period of remission (often thalidomide, corticosteroids, or both). Such maintenance therapy is designed to prolong the remission period—and there is some evidence that it may do so. However, there is no evidence that such therapy improves the overall survival of patients, and it may be associated with adverse effects.

Once the myeloma relapses, additional therapy can usually be administered. Many different agents can be effective here—thalidomide or bortezomib (Velcade) are often introduced at this stage. However, both the chance of obtaining a remission and the duration of the remission decrease with each successive relapse episode.

Selected patients are offered an allogeneic stem cell transplant. This approach provides a form of immuno-therapy against the myeloma and may be used imme-diately upon recovery from HDC-ASCS (sometimes referred to as a "tandem auto-allo transplant") or upon relapse of the disease. Allogeneic transplants are the only known treatments that have a potential for curing myeloma (see Questions 37 and 65–78).

JWH: While it is true that an allogeneic or mini-allogeneic transplant is the only known treatment that has a poten-tial for curing myeloma today, do not lose heart if you are unable to get such treatment yourself. Many of the thera-pies mentioned here can provide good response for many months or even years. Much is being done in myeloma research, and many doctors I have spoken with who are involved in treating myeloma are optimistic that new therapies will be found that will make myeloma much more treatable in the not too distant future.

34. What is a clinical trial, and how does it differ from the "standard of care"?

Clinical trials are performed in order to evaluate newer therapies and to compare the results of the newer therapies to standard treatment. New treat-ments are developed because scientists and doctors believe that they may be better than the current best standard therapy (**standard of care**). However, such new therapies can be proven to be superior only by performing clinical trials of the therapy.

Clinical trials can be of several different types known as **phases**. Promising new treatments are usually first identified through *preclinical* studies in the test tube or

Clinical trial

a research study designed to assess the effectiveness and/or safety of a newer or different treatment compared to the current stan-dard of care. This is the method whereby advances in cancer treatment occur.

Standard of care

a term used to describe the best cur-rent option for treat-ing a disease, based upon the results of previous clinical trials.

Phase

an indication of the type of clinical trial being performed. Phase I studies are among the earliest types of clinical trial. They are conducted using a new therapy and usually need only a small number of patients. Phase III trials are large, randomized compar-isons of a new ther-apy against the current standard of care.

on experimental animals. Once such a treatment is identified, it is first tested in humans in a **Phase I trial**. If the new treatment is a drug, this phase often (but not always) involves starting at lower doses of the drug and escalating (increasing) the administered dose in successive groups of patients. Such a trial establishes a safe dose for the drug and provides preliminary indication of the activity of the treatment. Once a successful Phase I trial is completed, the activity of the treatment is assessed in more detail in a **Phase II trial**. Treatments found to be active and safe in a Phase II study can then be formally compared to the current standard treatment (standard of care) in a **Phase III trial**. Phase III trials are usually much larger than Phase II trials, often involving several hundred patients or more. Also, Phase III trials contain at least two treatment options (also known as arms), one involving the new treatment (experimental arm) and one consisting of the best current standard treatment (control or standard arm).

In a Phase III trial, patients are assigned to receive either the new treatment or the standard treatment by a method akin to a flip of a coin. Neither the patient nor the physician gets to choose which treatment arm the patient is assigned to. Usually a computer decides the assignment, in a process known as randomization. Although some patients may be reluctant to participate if they are unable to choose exactly which treatment they receive, it is important to remember that Phase III trials are the most carefully designed and scrutinized of clinical trials. Patients receive at least the best standard therapy (which they would receive anyway if they elected to not participate in a clinical trial), and the newer (experimental) therapy is usually not available outside the clinical trial. Also, the information obtained

Treatment Options

Preclinical

experimental use of a drug in animals or test-tubes, before trials in humans are conducted.

Phase I trial

early study of a treatment designed to find best dose to use and assess initial side-effects in patients.

Phase II trial

a study of a treatment already shown to be relatively safe, designed to determine its activity against the disease.

Phase III trial

a large clinical trial formally comparing a new therapy against the best standard treatment available.

from a Phase III trial is essential if standard treatment is to be improved for the future.

The treatment administered in all clinical trials is carefully monitored by an institutional review board to ensure that it is an appropriate option for the patients to whom it is offered. When you participate in a clinical trial, the trial is usually explained to you by the physician who is conducting it. You are then given a consent form, which contains a description of the trial and the potential benefits and possible risks of participation, given in layman's terms. It is important that you carefully read the entire form and ask your physician to clarify anything that may not be clear in it before you sign. If you participate, your physician will administer treatment and follow-up assessments and tests in accordance with the written protocol of the trial.

35. Should I participate in a clinical trial?

Participation in a clinical trial is usually beneficial to both you and to patients with myeloma who are diagnosed and treated after you. You benefit because it may enable you to access a newer, cutting-edge form of therapy. Often this therapy will not be accessible to those not participating in the clinical trial. Also, patients treated in a clinical trial are usually monitored more rigorously than patients treated with standard therapy. Future patients will benefit from your participation in a clinical trial because you will be helping to establish the standard therapy of the future. The current standard treatment for any disease became established because of previously completed clinical trials. Studies have demonstrated that on average, cancer patients who participate in clinical trials do better than patients not treated in a clinical trial.

There are a few potential disadvantages to participating in a clinical trial. If the trial is not available locally, you may have to face the inconvenience of traveling to a center where such a trial is available. In addition, your oncologist is usually not free to change your treatment if it does not adhere to the protocol of the clinical trial. (This is not a major disadvantage, as the trial is usually designed by experts and includes options within the protocol if your condition changes. You can also always end your participation in the trial if your condition necessitates it.) The treatment being tested is new and therefore by definition does not have the track record of standard therapy. This means that the treatment can sometimes turn out to be less effective than anticipated, and unexpected side effects can sometimes come to light during the trial.

In general, however, the benefits of participating in a clinical trial outweigh the potential disadvantages.

36. I was not eligible for a clinical trial of a newer treatment I am interested in. Is there another mechanism for accessing the drug?

Experimental drugs or treatments that are not approved for clinical use by the Food and Drug Administration can usually be accessed only through a clinical trial for which you are eligible. However, sometimes there is a "compassionate use" program that provides nonresearch access to an experimental agent.

Such a program may or may not be in place for the treatment you are interested in. If such a program is in place, it is usually administered by the sponsor of the clinical trial using that agent (this is usually the company making the treatment, although in some cases it can be a branch of the National Cancer Institute). Generally, the following criteria apply for accessing a treatment or drug through a compassionate use program: (1) You must have failed standard therapies for the disease, (2) there must already be evidence from clinical trials showing that the treatment is active for your type of myeloma, (3) you must be ineligible for available clinical trials of the treatment, and (4) your doctor must determine that you are likely to benefit from the drug.

Your oncologist can find out whether such a program is available for the treatment you are interested in.

37. Is myeloma curable?

Myeloma has traditionally been considered an incurable disease. Typically, patients with myeloma respond well to initial therapy. The majority of patients achieve at least some objective response to the initial treatment regimen used. However, a complete remission is achieved by only a small minority, and in almost all patients, the disease does relapse at some time following completion of the initial treatment regimen. This can be a few months to a few years later, depending upon the aggressiveness of the patient's myeloma, the stage of the disease when it was first treated, and the type of treatment received. Some evidence exists to suggest that patients who receive an autologous stem cell transplant immediately after initial treatment remain free of the disease longer and even survive longer than patients who do not receive an autologous stem cell transplant as part of their initial therapy. However, almost all patients—including those who have received an autologous transplant—will eventually relapse.

Once the disease relapses, it may remain responsive to treatment. The treatment given after a relapse is often different from the one given as initial therapy. However, with each successive relapse the remission achieved is usually shorter, until the myeloma becomes resistant to available therapies and/or the patient cannot tolerate further therapy because of accumulated side effects such as neuropathy. Some elderly patients with myeloma may, of course, die from an unrelated condition before their myeloma becomes resistant to therapy. However, the majority of patients in the past have died of myeloma that is resistant to further treatment. It is possible that some newer therapies may change this prospect. However, none of the currently approved or experimental treatments for full-blown myeloma other than allogeneic stem cell transplantation have been shown to cure the disease.

Allogeneic stem cell transplantation (see Question 68) is the only known therapy that shows a clear potential to cure patients with multiple myeloma. Some patients who have undergone an allogeneic transplant are free of any sign of relapse 5 to 15 years later. In contrast, patients treated with standard therapies very rarely stay in remission for 5 years. It is felt that allogeneic transplantation can cure myeloma because it allows the patient's immune system to be replaced by that of the donor, allowing the donor's immune cells to mount an immune attack upon the myeloma cells. However, allogeneic transplantation has traditionally been an option for only a minority of patients with myeloma. A matched donor is necessary, and the patient has had to be relatively young and in excellent general health. Even in patients who meet these criteria, the procedure is complex and has a significant risk of treatment-related complications, which may in some cases be fatal. That is why this type of transplant has not been offered to all patients with myeloma.

Technological advances in allogeneic transplantation over the last 5 years are making the procedure safer and may therefore make it a possibility even for some older and less healthy patients with myeloma. The use of nonablative or "mini-transplants" is among the most significant advances in this area. However, allogeneic transplantation remains more complicated and more risky than other treatments for myeloma, and the decision to proceed with an allogeneic transplant must be made with a full understanding of the procedure, its possible benefits, and potential risks.

38. I have been in complete remission for 5 years. Can I consider myself cured?

The duration of response to treatment is highly variable in myeloma patients. Although the overwhelming majority of patients treated with standard therapy will experience disease relapse within 5 years, a small fraction may have more prolonged responses. However, an eventual relapse is still very likely. Patients who have undergone an allogeneic stem cell transplant may in some cases be cured if their disease has not recurred after 5 years, but here too, further follow-up is necessary.

39. What is chemotherapy?

Although **chemotherapy** can be strictly defined as using a chemical to treat a disease, the term is commonly used to mean a drug that treats cancer by attacking cells in the body that are dividing. Because cancer cells must divide for the cancer to grow, and they usually divide more rapidly than normal cells, blocking cell division or killing cells that are dividing can be very beneficial in cancer therapy. Indeed, chemotherapy has been the mainstay of treatment for most advanced cancers. However, cell division also occurs in most normal organs of the body in order to replace cells that age and die naturally. Thus, chemotherapy can have side effects because it also acts upon normal organs, especially those with a high cell turnover, such as the bone marrow or gut.

Cancer cells are usually slower to recover from the effects of chemotherapy than normal cells, and therefore chemotherapy is often given in **cycles**, meaning that the drug is given followed by an interval (usually 2 to 4 weeks), after which it is administered again. Normal cells recover during the interval period, but cancer cells do not recover completely, allowing a progressive reduction in the number of cancer cells in the body with repeated cycles.

40. What are corticosteroids?

Corticosteroids (sometimes known as glucocorticoids) are drugs that are similar to normal body hormones that regulate your body's metabolism, appetite, ability to mount inflammatory and immune responses, and so forth. Although different from chemotherapy drugs in the traditional sense (see Question 39), these

Chemotherapy

the treatment of cancer using drugs or chemicals. The term is usually used to refer more specifically to drugs or chemicals that preferentially kill dividing cells.

Cycle (of treatment)

a defined treatment period that is repeated several times in order to complete the course of therapy.

Corticosteroids

drugs chemically related to normal body hormones that control metabolism and inflammation.

Treatment Options

drugs, which are often taken orally, are active against myeloma and some other cancers of the bone marrow and lymph nodes. Dexamethasone (Decadron) and prednisone are the two corticosteroids most commonly used to treat myeloma. These drugs are often used in combination with chemotherapy and other drugs (such as in the VAD, M&P, and TD regimens described in Question 33), but they can also be used alone.

Unlike chemotherapy drugs, corticosteroids do not suppress bone marrow function. This means that they do not by themselves cause your blood counts to go down. Although these drugs are sometimes just called "steroids" by physicians and patients, they are quite different from anabolic steroids, the drugs that athletes sometimes abuse. Unlike anabolic steroids, corticosteroids do not promote muscle growth but in fact cause a loss of muscle tissue.

Among other side effects, corticosteroids can raise blood sugar and blood pressure, thin the bones, weaken the immune system, and cause joint problems. These side effects are particularly problematic if the drugs are used in high doses for prolonged periods of time. When used in intermittent "pulses" for short periods, these drugs are very useful in the treatment of myeloma.

41. What are Aredia and Zometa?

One of the most significant effects of myeloma on the body is a severe thinning of the bone in areas next to the parts of the bone marrow that are most severely involved. This can lead to bone fractures that occur with minimal or no trauma (pathological fractures), which in turn lead to severe pain and an impaired ability to move and function. These fractures most commonly occur when the myeloma involves weight-bearing bones (such as those in the spine or legs). Thinning of the bone also releases calcium, which is normally bound to bone, into the bloodstream. This can cause an increase in blood calcium (hypercalcemia), which in turn causes dehydration, mental confusion, constipation, and renal failure.

Palmidronate disodium (Aredia) and zoledronic acid (Zometa) belong to a group of drugs known as **bisphosphonates**, which are used to prevent and treat bone disease caused by myeloma. In patients with myeloma, intravenous bisphosphonates delay and reduce the number of bone complications (such as fractures, radiation therapy to bone, surgery to bone, or spinal cord compression) and decrease bone pain. They also normalize levels of calcium in patients with increased blood calcium. These drugs are given by injection approximately every month to myeloma patients with bone disease visible on an x-ray or with general bone thinning. Once started they should probably be continued indefinitely, unless the risks and side effects of treatment outweigh the perceived benefits. Patients should be monitored for kidney dysfunction with blood tests prior to starting on these drugs, and at least every 3 to 6 months while on these drugs.

In test-tube and animal experiments, some bisphosphonates exerted direct effects against myeloma cells independent of their effect against bone loss. It is unclear whether this mechanism also benefits patients with myeloma who are treated with these drugs.

Bisphosphonates
drugs used to prevent and treat bone disease caused by myeloma.

42. What is thalidomide?

Thalidomide is an oral drug that has been shown to be very effective at treating myeloma. This drug was originally developed as a treatment for morning sickness and was used for that purpose in the 1950s and '60s. However, its use for that condition was abandoned when it was discovered that the drug can result in severe birth defects when used early in pregnancy. Thalidomide is approved in the United States for the treatment of symptoms that develop in some people with leprosy (an infectious disease found more commonly in developing countries). It is not as yet approved by the FDA specifically for the treatment of myeloma.

Exactly how thalidomide works against myeloma is uncertain. However, this drug has several biologic effects that may contribute to its activity:

- It decreases the availability of chemical messages (cytokines) that are vital for the growth and survival of myeloma cells.
- It may stimulate the body's immune system to fight myeloma.
- It inhibits the formation of new blood vessels that are necessary for the growth of myeloma cells.
- It inhibits the adhesion of myeloma cells to the "scaffolding" of the bone marrow (stromal cells).

Thalidomide is a relatively safe drug as long as it is not used by pregnant women. However, it does have several side effects, which can limit the ability of some patients with myeloma to tolerate it. Specifically, thalidomide can cause drowsiness; constipation; nerve damage (peripheral neuropathy), which can result in numbness and pain in the limbs; fatigue; and an increased tendency to clot formation in the blood vessels. Generally, the severity of these side effects is related to the dose of the drug used. As thalidomide can be active at low doses, it is customary for the physician to start you at a low dose (50–100 mg) once a day and then to increase the dose only if no limiting side effects occur.

The peripheral neuropathy from this drug can be cumulative (can add up over time) and may even affect your ability to tolerate other antimyeloma drugs, such as Velcade (see Question 44), later in the course of your disease. Although the neuropathy may improve after the drug is discontinued, cases that are more advanced may not be completely reversible even when the patient stops taking thalidomide. It is therefore important to be aware of symptoms such as increasing numbness or pain in the arms or legs and to make your physician aware of these. Question 61 discusses peripheral neuropathy further.

Combining thalidomide and corticosteroid drugs (see Question 40) increases the potential risk of blood clots. You should discuss measures that can minimize this risk if you are treated with this combination. Because of the risks of severe birth defects if pregnant women are exposed to thalidomide, routine pregnancy testing is necessary if women of childbearing age are treated. Participation in the System for Thalidomide Education and Prescribing Safety (STEPS) program is also required. The patient must also sign a consent form before treatment with thalidomide can begin.

Thalidomide has been shown to be effective in treating advanced myeloma that has relapsed after other treatments. Therefore, most oncologists use this drug when the disease has relapsed, either by itself or in combination with another antimyeloma drug such as dexamethasone. Studies have also shown that thalidomide can be effective in initial therapy (where it is usually given as part of a combination regimen with other drugs) and as a maintenance treatment in patients who have already achieved remission with another treatment regimen.

JWH: Thalidomide is a very interesting drug, and it seems to be effective against myeloma for a time. I know many people who have taken it, and in fact I took it myself for 6 months. It reduced the amount of myeloma in my system, and the side effects were very tolerable. It helped me get to the point where I could receive a mini-allogeneic transplant. I do agree that neuropathy is a problem. In my limited experience, it is a major reason that people stop taking it. I have numbness on the soles of my feet just from taking the drug for 6 months. Others I know say they can't feel anything up to their mid-calves because of the neuropathy. Just be aware that there is a trade-off.

43. What are the ImiDs?

ImiD

immunomodulatory molecule. Refers to compounds related to thalidomide that may stimulate the immune response against cancer in addition to other activities.

ImiD is the abbreviation for immunomodulatory drug. The term is used specifically to describe drugs taken orally that are structurally related to thalidomide. These drugs have been developed to be somewhat more potent than thalidomide and to lack, or to show a diminished tendency to develop, some of the bothersome side effects of thalidomide. Currently these drugs are not approved by the FDA for use in treating myeloma; they are available only in clinical trials. Two main compounds are being tested against myeloma: Revlimid (CC-5013) and Actimid (CC-4047). Both have been shown to be effective against myeloma in reported studies. However, direct comparisons with thalidomide have not yet been reported, and thus it is not yet certain whether the ImiDs will prove more effective than thalidomide in treating myeloma patients. These drugs seem to have a reduced incidence of the side effects commonly associated with thalidomide, especially peripheral neuropathy, drowsiness, and constipation. However, they may cause more suppression of bone marrow function than is usual with thalidomide.

44. What is Velcade?

Velcade (also known as bortezomib) is a new drug approved in the United States to treat myeloma that has relapsed or is refractory after at least two prior treatments. It belongs to a completely new class of drugs known as **proteasome inhibitors**. This drug acts differently from traditional chemotherapy drugs and appears to be active against myeloma and several other cancers. It is administered as an intravenous injection, usually given twice a week for four injections followed by a 10-day rest period before the cycle is repeated.

Proteasome inhibitors

a completely new class of biologic agent that act by inhibiting the proteasome–a mechanism by which cell proteins are eliminated from cells.

One of the major side effects of the drug is peripheral neuropathy (numbness, tingling, and pain in the arms and legs—see Question 61). This problem can usually be reversed if it is detected early and either the drug is stopped or the dose is reduced. However, some patients may not completely recover, and those who have already developed neuropathy or other drugs that can cause nerve damage are at increased risk of neuropathy due to Velcade. Other side effects of Velcade include stomach upset or diarrhea, fatigue, a low platelet count, and fevers.

Although Velcade is usually used alone to treat relapsed myeloma, dexamethasone can be added for patients who do not have an optimal response. The use of Velcade in the initial treatment of myeloma, and its use in combination with other agents, is currently being explored in clinical trials.

45. What is radiation therapy, and when is it used against myeloma?

Radiation therapy
the use of x-rays to treat cancer.

Radiation therapy involves the use of x-rays to treat cancer. Usually, x-rays from an external source are directed at a part of the body involved with the disease. The treatment is delivered in "fractions" usually given once a day 5 days per week (occasionally the fractions are administered more frequently). Myeloma cells are usually highly sensitive to radiation therapy, and this treatment is highly effective against disease that is either localized or causing symptoms only at a localized site. Radiation therapy is used against myeloma mainly to relieve symptoms that are localized, such as localized bone pain, spinal cord compression, and localized involvement of a weight-bearing bone that is at risk of imminent fracture.

Radiation does not have many of the general side effects of chemotherapy, but it can have some disadvantages: Daily visits to the radiation therapy department are usually needed. If part of the gut is also irradiated, there can be nausea, vomiting, diarrhea, and throat pain. If extensive portions of the spine and/or pelvis are irradiated, bone marrow function within the irradiated areas will be severely impaired, leading to possible difficulty in tolerating subsequent chemotherapy and in collecting stem cells for autologous transplantation.

46. Is surgery useful in treating myeloma?

Surgery is not commonly used to treat myeloma. It is sometimes used instead of or in addition to radiation therapy to treat spinal cord compression, which can be a medical emergency in myeloma patients. Orthopedic surgeons can sometimes stabilize a bony structure that is weakened by myeloma by inserting metal rods or other supporting structures into it.

47. What are vertebroplasty and kyphoplasty, and how can they help?

Vertebroplasty and **kyphoplasty** are relatively new procedures designed to relieve symptoms and improve quality of life in patients with myeloma who develop compression fractures of the spine. Weakening of the vertebral bodies in the spine caused by myeloma results in these bones collapsing on top of themselves. This in turn leads to pain, loss of height, and a stooped posture, which impairs patients' ability to function and negatively affects their quality of life.

Both vertebroplasty and kyphoplasty help relieve these problems through the injection of a cementlike substance into the fractured bone. A needle is inserted into the bone under x-ray guidance, and the liquid cement is then injected into the bony space. The procedure is usually performed under local anesthesia, but general anesthetic may occasionally be needed. As the cementlike material hardens, the bone is strengthened.

For kyphoplasty, an additional attempt is made to expand the vertebral body in order to regain some of the height that has been lost due to the fracture. This is done by inserting a balloon into the bony cavity. The

Treatment Options

Vertebroplasty

a procedure in which a cementlike substance is injected into a collapsed spinal bone in order to re-expand it and thus relieve pain and loss of height.

Kyphoplasty

a procedure to treat the pain of spinal compression fractures by injection of cement-like substance into the bone.

balloon is then expanded to the required height, and a cementlike substance is inserted into it. By expanding the bone and restoring height, kyphoplasty realigns the bony structures, resulting in relief from pain and improvement of posture in the patient. The procedure is usually performed by either a surgeon or an interventional radiologist. In experienced hands, it involves minimal risk—very rarely, leakage of the cement outside the bone can occur. This usually does not cause any symptoms. You should consider these procedures if you have back pain or limitation of activity associated with compression fractures of the spine.

48. How is bone pain managed in myeloma patients?

Bone pain is a common symptom associated with myeloma. There are several different causes of bone pain in myeloma. Actively growing myeloma cells in the marrow and surrounding bone can cause pain directly or through the release of chemical messengers. Alternatively, myeloma can sometimes extend outside the bone and can impinge upon nerve roots or the spine, which can also cause bone pain. Bone pain in myeloma patients may also result from spinal or other fractures, which then lead to misalignment of the bone and pressure upon nerves. Patients with myeloma-associated bone pain usually notice significant improvement in their pain as well as in their ability to function once their myeloma responds to treatment. However, bone pain due to misalignment resulting from a fracture may not respond completely to treatment even if the myeloma itself responds to treatment. In this situation, vertebroplasty (see Question 47) and other surgical procedures may be of benefit.

Patients with bone pain related to myeloma are usually treated with strong analgesic medications (painkillers). When these are used, the physician will usually prescribe a long-acting form of painkiller designed to prevent pain. This avoids the need for the patient to feel pain in order to receive the medication. Although a short-acting painkiller is also prescribed simultaneously, it is intended to be used only if the pain manages to break through the long-acting painkiller and should not be primarily relied upon for control of the pain. The objective is to use as much long-acting pain medication as necessary to fully suppress the patient's pain so that the short-acting medication is either not necessary or minimally used.

49. Why does kidney failure occur in myeloma, and how is it treated?

Impairment of kidney function is one of the most common complications of myeloma. Approximately one quarter to one third of all myeloma patients will have kidney problems during the course of their illness, and about 10% of patients will have severe kidney failure when their myeloma is diagnosed. Kidney failure in myeloma is most commonly due to myeloma protein being deposited in the kidney tubules and is particularly common in cases in which the myeloma cells produce only a light-chain protein. However, other factors related to myeloma, such as dehydration, high blood calcium, infection, medications, and amyloidosis (see Question 5), can also contribute.

Symptoms of kidney failure include loss of appetite with nausea and vomiting, diarrhea, fatigue, and drowsiness. If untreated, the kidney failure itself can be fatal. Patients with severe kidney failure often require dialysis. The kidney function often improves significantly upon treatment of the myeloma and can return to normal. However, some patients are left with chronic kidney dysfunction and may even require long-term dialysis.

The presence of kidney failure may make it difficult to use some chemotherapy agents that are normally excreted through the kidney. In patients with myeloma, kidney failure can be prevented by adequate hydration, treatment of infections, and avoidance of medications that damage the kidneys.

JWH: I was one of those who had total kidney failure when first diagnosed. I needed dialysis for 3 months. There was some doubt that I would ever get my kidney function back, but I did. My kidneys responded beautifully once I began myeloma treatment, and they have been doing fine ever since. If you have kidney difficulties because of myeloma, do not assume that your kidney failure is permanent. Your problems may last for only a few weeks or months.

50. Is there a role for alternative/ complementary therapies in myeloma?

Maintaining a healthy lifestyle is part of the general approach to fighting myeloma. This includes a healthy diet and a reasonable aerobic exercise regimen. Weight-training exercise can be hazardous in patients with myeloma bone disease. Whereas measures like acupuncture may be of benefit in myeloma, as they can be in other conditions associated with pain, most alternative/complementary measures have not been rigorously tested in myeloma. Therefore, while some may be of benefit, others may potentially be harmful. It is important that you consider nontraditional therapies as an adjunct to and not a replacement for proven conventional treatment approaches. If you are planning to receive any nontraditional therapies, it important that you fully discuss these and any potential effects on your myeloma with your oncologist.

JWH: Alternative therapies are something you should consider, but, as was just stated, not instead of conventional therapies. I strongly suggest, for example, that you consult with a nutritionist who is knowledgeable in helping with cancer. I have consulted with a nutritionist for quite a while now, and I believe his suggestions have been of benefit. It is true that few studies can substantiate the benefits of alternative therapies, but to be frank, some of that is because conventional medicine doesn't study them. When you're diagnosed with myeloma, and you have heard from a source that a particular treatment is very effective, it is hard to sort out whether you should heed the advice or ignore it, and your oncologist will likely say, "There aren't any studies that prove that treatment to be effective."

Let me give an example. When I consulted with my nutritionist, he told me to start taking curcumin. It is an herb, or food supplement, that is widely available and widely claimed by nutritionists to be an effective treatment against many cancers. I began to take curcumin, and I continue to do so. Over a year later there was an article in Blood, *the magazine of hematology. It reported on a study that showed curcumin to be effective against myeloma (at least in test-tube studies). Nonetheless, doctors still don't recommend taking it because there have been no Phase III studies confirming its efficacy in humans. True enough—but it still might be effective.*

When you're a patient looking for help, waiting for studies to be completed is unsatisfactory. You may decide that curcumin is worth trying after consulting your physician and a nutritionist. There are similar alternatives to consider as well. I mention these not to disagree with the usual medical recommendations, but rather to point out that doctors simply don't recommend treatments that haven't been proven to be effective under very rigorous standards. As a patient, you may want to explore other options that have not yet been proved by studies. We have to look at things practically and seek help where we can find it.

51. Is there a vaccine therapy for myeloma?

Vaccination involves the injection or administration of a special preparation designed to elicit an active immune response against at least one ingredient in that preparation. As you are aware, vaccination is used most successfully to prevent infectious disease. This is because the vaccine allows the body to mount an immune response against an infectious agent even before one has been exposed to it.

Researchers are exploring whether similar vaccine therapies can be effective against cancer. Some researchers have tried to use the abnormal M-protein in myeloma as a vaccine. This is done by purifying the protein and then injecting it with chemicals known as adjuvants, which are known to stimulate immune responses. Such vaccine therapies have been tested in clinical trials on myeloma patients. It is not presently clear whether they improve outcomes in myeloma, and vaccine therapy is not approved by the Food and Drug Administration for use in myeloma. You may be able to participate in a clinical trial of vaccine therapy for myeloma.

52. What is a central venous catheter, and who needs it?

Many treatments used for myeloma are administered into a vein (i.v. therapy). While many of these medications can be administered into a peripheral vein, repeated infusion into the peripheral veins of the arms eventually leads to hardening and loss of the available veins. Also, some of the treatments used, such as adriamycin and vincristine are **vesicant** drugs, meaning that they can cause severe tissue damage if they leak out of the vein due to a poorly positioned catheter.

To avoid these problems and to make it easier to administer these drugs by prolonged infusion, many patients have a **central venous catheter** (sometimes called a central line) inserted. The end of this catheter is placed into one of the large veins in the chest (close to the heart), and the other end is often tunneled through the skin and ends in a reservoir under the skin, which can be accessed with a needle. This type of catheter is known as an implantable port or portacath. Another type of central venous catheter, known as a Hickman or Groshong catheter, comes out through the skin of the chest and extends a few inches away from the skin. In each case, these catheters can stay in place for many months but require care to prevent infection. They also require flushing to prevent clots from forming within them. The frequency of flushing depends on the type of catheter and can vary from daily to once a month. You or a family member can be

Vesicant

a type of drug that causes severe tissue damage if it leaks out from the veins into the tissues surrounding it.

Central venous catheter

a catheter placed into one of the body's large central veins (such as the large veins in the neck or shoulder region).

taught to flush and dress the catheter. A wider-bore version of the Hickman catheter is often used for stem cell collection (see Question 67).

Sometimes a more temporary form of central venous catheter is inserted by threading it up from one of the veins in the arm. This type is known as a percutaneously inserted central catheter, or PICC. It is a smaller catheter and can be placed quickly by nurses without the need for a physician.

53. What problems can result from the presence of a central venous catheter?

Occasionally problems can occur during the insertion of a catheter. These include unexpected bleeding or a puncture of the lining of the lung, causing a pneumothorax (air that collects between the lung and chest wall). In experienced hands these problems are rare and can be managed with appropriate intervention. A chest x-ray is usually performed after a catheter is inserted to look for an occult pneumothorax.

Common problems that develop while a catheter is in place include infection of the catheter site and a blood clot in the vein where the catheter is inserted. Infection can often be managed by using antibiotics while leaving the catheter in place. However, serious infections may require the removal of the catheter. A clot around the catheter is usually treated with medications such as coumadin that thin the blood and help the clot dissolve.

Central catheters are very useful to the patient because they make repeated access of the peripheral veins unnecessary, and they can also be used for blood draws. In most cases, the complications just described can be avoided by adequate care of the catheter.

54. How do I know whether my treatment is working?

When you receive treatment for myeloma, your oncologist will assess the response of your disease to the therapy he or she is prescribing. This assessment should be performed on a regular basis (for example, every 2 cycles or every 2 months of therapy). To assess response, your oncologist will repeat some or all of the tests that were initially performed when your myeloma was diagnosed. If the myeloma protein (M-protein) was easily detectable in your blood at diagnosis, this is one of the best tests to use to determine the response. The level of the myeloma protein can be measured in one of two ways: (1) the total level of the immunoglobulins in the blood can be measured with a QIG test (see Question 15). If the IgG or IgA level was much above normal prior to treatment, a fall in this level will indicate a response. (2) The SPEP test (see Question 13) can be repeated. This test measures the M-protein band by assessing its size after running blood serum through a gel under an electric current.

Less frequently, your oncologist will repeat the bone marrow biopsy and skeletal survey. In patients with light-chain-only myeloma, the amount of M-protein excreted in the urine in a 24-hour period is one of the best ways to measure response. In patients with myeloma that is nonsecretory (one that does not make a measurable M-protein), response assessment can be more difficult. Here the percentage of plasma cells is often used as a surrogate measure of response. However, the bone marrow biopsy results can be patchy and are clearly not as quantitative as blood protein measurement. In these cases it is worth performing a free-light-chain assay (see Question 17) to see whether small quantities of otherwise undetectable light-chain production by these myelomas can be detected.

55. What are the different types of response my myeloma can have to treatment?

Based upon clinical evaluation and the tests mentioned in Question 54, your oncologist will try to define the type of response you have had to the therapy. By defining the response using standard criteria that other oncologists also use, he or she will be able to judge the success of the treatment and will know whether it is necessary to use a different therapy. Your response to treatment can also help determine your prognosis. Doctors who treat myeloma use several standard categories of response. These are defined in Table 4.

Table 4   Standard Categories of Response to Myeloma Treatment

Treatment Response*	Definition
Cure	Complete eradication of the myeloma with no possibility of recurrence. No evidence remains of the disease.
Complete response (CR)	No detectable M-protein in the blood or urine (using immunofixation) and normal percentage of plasma cells in the bone marrow (< 5%).
Very good partial response (or near complete response) (VGPR)	Greater than 90% decrease in M-protein.
Partial response (PR)	Greater than 50% decrease in M-protein.
Minor response (or minimal response) (MR)	Less than 25–50% decrease in M-protein.
Stable disease (SD)	Stable disease parameters (including number and extent of bone abnormalities) with no greater than 25% change in M-protein.
Progressive disease (PD)	Greater than 25% increase in M-protein, new bony lesions, or a new plasmacytoma.

*Response may also be called remission.

TABLE 5   Drugs Used in the Treatment of Myeloma and Associated Disease

Type	Generic Name	Brand Name	Manufacturer
Chemotherapy	Vincristine	Oncovin	Lilly
Chemotherapy	Doxorubicin	Adriamycin	Pharmacia
Chemotherapy	Liposomal doxorubicin	Doxil	Alza
Chemotherapy	Melphalan	Alkeran	Glaxo-SmithKline
Chemotherapy	Cyclophosphamide	Cytoxan	Mead Johnson/ Bristol-Myers Squibb
Chemotherapy	Chlorambucil	Leukeran	Glaxo-Smithkline
Chemotherapy	Carmustine	BiCNU	Mead Johnson/ Bristol-Myers Squibb
Chemotherapy	Cisplatin	Platinol	Bristol-Myers Squibb
Chemotherapy	Etoposide	Vepesid	Mead Johnson/ Bristol-Myers Squibb
Coricosteroid	Prednisone	Deltasone	Pharmacia
Coricosteroid	Dexamethasone	Decadron	Merck
Proteasome Inhibitor	Bortezomib	Velcade	Millennium
Immuno-modulator/ anti-angio-genesis/multiple mechanisms	Thalidomide	Thalomid	Celgene
Biologic	Arsenic trioxide	Trisenox	Cell Therapeutics Inc.
Biologic	Alpha-interferon	Roferon; Intron-A	Roche Schering
Antibiotic	Clarithromycin	Biaxin	Abbott
Bisphosphonate	Pamidronate disodium	Aredia	Novartis
Bisphosphonate	Zoledronic acid	Zometa	Novartis
Growth factor	Erythropoietin alfa	Procrit	Ortho-Biotech
Growth factor	Darbepoetin	Aranesp	Amgen
Growth factor	Filgrastim (G-CSF)	Neupogen	Amgen
Growth factor	Pegfilgrastim	Neulasta	Amgen

In most studies, the better the response achieved, the better the patient's prognosis for survival. A complete response or CR is achieved in only a minority of patients with conventional therapy.

In many patients, a partial response is achieved (VGPR, PR, or MR), and there is then no further response with additional cycles of treatment. This state is sometimes called the plateau phase. There is usually no value in continuing the same treatment after a plateau phase is achieved.

PART FOUR

Side Effects and Complications of Treatment

What are the main side effects of chemotherapy?

What precautions are necessary if my white blood cell (WBC) count is low because of chemotherapy?

My platelet count is low because of chemotherapy. What does that mean?

More . . .

56. What are the main side effects of chemotherapy?

Although most patients think of nausea and vomiting as one of the most common side effects of chemotherapy, the actual incidence of severe nausea and vomiting is now quite small due to the availability and use of strong medications that prevent this problem if given with chemotherapy. Sometimes additional medication is necessary following the chemotherapy to prevent delayed nausea and vomiting. The actual incidence of chemotherapy-induced nausea and vomiting varies depending upon the regimen used, the age of the patient, and so on. However, fear of this side effect is no longer justified because most patients experience either no nausea or mild symptoms.

Hair loss is a common side effect of some chemotherapy regimens. Adriamycin, used as part of the VAD regimen, and higher doses of melphalan, are particularly prone to cause hair loss. The degree of hair loss can be variable, and for most patients it is temporary, with hair growth resuming some weeks or months after the discontinuation of chemotherapy. Although many patients are comfortable with the temporary change in their appearance, some patients benefit from the use of a wig or head coverings during this period. Many of the agents used to treat myeloma are not associated with major hair loss; these include corticosteroids, thalidomide, and Velcade.

Most traditional chemotherapy agents cause a temporary but significant suppression of the function of normal cells in the bone marrow. This results in low blood counts, including a low blood hemoglobin, low white blood cell count, and low blood platelet count that may last for days to weeks between cycles of chemotherapy. These low blood counts can in turn cause fatigue and make a patient more susceptible to infections and bleeding. These side effects are discussed in Questions 57 through 59 below. Your oncologist will monitor your blood counts when you receive chemotherapy and will make adjustments to your treatment as necessary.

Some chemotherapy agents seem to deplete the number and quality of stem cells present in the bone marrow. When used for many cycles, these agents can lead to chronically low blood counts, can impair your ability to tolerate further chemotherapy, and can make it difficult for your physician to collect stem cells for autologous transplantation (see Question 68). Melphalan and BiCNU are among the agents most likely to cause this effect, especially when used for longer than 6 months. Their prolonged use is therefore now discouraged in patients who are candidates for autologous transplantation.

A low blood platelet count can also result from Velcade therapy. Thalidomide and corticosteroids usually do not have severe effects upon blood counts. However, corticosteroids can cause a patient to be susceptible to infections by suppressing the immune system in other ways.

Peripheral neuropathy is a side effect of vincristine, which is used in the VAD regimen. Administering vincristine by a slow infusion rather than by a rapid injection helps minimize this side effect. Peripheral neuropathy can be a major side effect of therapy with thalidomide and Velcade and is discussed in more detail in Question 61.

JWH: I have had personal experience with most of the chemotherapy drugs used in myeloma treatment. Like most people, when told I had to undergo chemotherapy, I was afraid of nausea and hair loss. The first chemotherapy drug I received was melphalan. I had a lot of nausea because I was not given antinausea medication before I received the treatment. If you are not offered antinausea medication before chemotherapy, you might want to ask for it. With those medications, the other times I was given chemotherapy were unremarkable. I noticed some fatigue, and some of the treatments caused my hair to fall out, but it grew back and I now look quite normal.

57. What precautions are necessary if my white blood cell (WBC) count is low because of chemotherapy?

Low WBC counts are a common and usually temporary side effect of chemotherapy for myeloma. In most cases, serious complications from the low blood counts that result from chemotherapy can be prevented by taking appropriate precautionary measures. Some white cells in the blood are called **neutrophils** and are important in fighting bacterial infection. They can ingest and kill bacteria and some other microbes that have managed to get into the body. Decreased levels of these cells increase the risk of potentially life-threatening infections, which can rapidly become overwhelming.

Neutrophil

the main type of white cell in the blood that fights against bacterial and fungal infections.

Your oncologist will arrange for regular checks of your CBC following chemotherapy. The absolute neutrophil count (ANC) can be worked out from the CBC by multiplying the WBC by the percentage of white cells that are neutrophils (also called granulocytes). Ideally, the ANC should be higher than 1500 cells/μL. The risk of serious bacterial infections increases significantly if the ANC is less than 500 cells/μL of blood and is very severe if the ANC is less than 100 cells/μL. Patients with a low ANC need to report any infection symptoms promptly to their physician so that antibiotic therapy can be started immediately. These symptoms may include fevers, chills, cough, and skin and mouth inflammation. In some cases your physician may choose to use antibiotics to prevent infections if your ANC is low (sometimes this is referred to as being **neutropenic**), even if there are no symptoms of an infection. Also, growth factor drug injections (e.g. Neupogen or Neulasta) may sometimes be given to increase your production of white blood cells and speed recovery of the ANC. These growth factor drugs stimulate the bone marrow to produce neutrophils and thus may shorten the period of neutropenia.

Neutropenia
an abnormally low concentration of neutrophils in the blood.

JWH: When your white blood cell count is low, and you are neutropenic, you will be told. You may be asked to wear a mask to prevent infection. It feels strange to wear a mask (I wore one on an airplane once), but it is worth it if it keeps you from getting a cold or infection that your immune system may not be able to fight off.

58. My platelet count is low because of chemotherapy. What does that mean?

Platelets are small cells that are normally present in large numbers in the blood (150,000–400,000/μL). These cells help form blood clots. Platelet levels are reduced below normal by several types of chemotherapy. A low blood platelet count may cause bleeding. If the platelet count is very low (below 10,000–20,000/μL), this risk is severe. Life-threatening bleeding (especially bleeding in the brain) can occur with minimal trauma or even spontaneously. Thus, your physician will monitor your platelet count after chemotherapy. It is important to minimize the risk of injury by avoiding contact sports, for example, when your platelet count is significantly below the lower limit of normal. If the platelet count falls below a specified value (usually 10,000/μL but possibly higher in certain circumstances), or if there are bleeding symptoms, your physician may arrange for a transfusion of platelets, which will temporarily increase the platelet count and decrease the risk of bleeding.

59. What causes anemia in myeloma patients, and how is it treated?

Hemoglobin is the protein present in red blood cells that makes blood look red. Its main function is to carry oxygen from the lungs to tissues where it is needed. Anemia is defined as a hemoglobin level in the blood that is below normal (normal levels are different for men and women). Anemia can cause fatigue, shortness of breath, dizziness, palpitations, and heart failure. Whether anemia causes any of these symptoms depends to some degree upon how suddenly it develops and how severe it is. There are many potential causes of anemia in myeloma patients. These include replacement of bone marrow function by myeloma cells, effects of chemotherapy, kidney failure, bleeding, infections, and so forth.

Anemia caused directly by the myeloma will to some degree respond to treatment of the myeloma. However, the treatments themselves, such as chemotherapy, can exacerbate anemia in the short term. Your physician will prescribe injections of a red blood cell growth hormone (either erythropoietin [Procrit] or darbepoetin [Aranesp]) to help alleviate this problem. Usually this hormone is given once a week or every other week as an injection. It can take several weeks to reach its maximal effect. If the anemia is very severe or does not respond to the growth factors, a blood transfusion may be necessary.

60. What causes fatigue during therapy for myeloma?

Fatigue is a very common complaint in patients receiving therapy for myeloma. There are many different potential causes of fatigue. Anemia resulting from myeloma or chemotherapy is a common and easily treated cause of fatigue (see Question 59). Some therapeutic agents can sometimes cause fatigue in patients who are not anemic. This is a complaint experienced by some patients on Velcade and on certain chemotherapy agents. In these cases the symptoms may sometimes be relieved by reducing the dose, administering the drug less frequently, or, if necessary, discontinuing the offending agent. Muscle weakness can be caused by corticosteroid therapy, which can in turn produce fatigue upon exertion. In some cases the pain and debilitation associated with advanced myeloma bone disease can result in deconditioning of the muscles and cardiovascular system caused by prolonged immobility. Such patients can experience significant fatigue, even after the pain is relieved by therapy. A graduated exercise regimen designed to recondition those organ systems will help relieve fatigue in such patients.

61. What is peripheral neuropathy, and how is it managed?

Peripheral nervous system

nerves that run from the brain and spinal cord to the rest of the body.

Peripheral neuropathy

disease of or damage to nerves outside the central nervous system (brain and spinal cord). Peripheral neuropathy can be sensory (causing numbness and pain) or motor (causing weakness or paralysis) or a mix of the two.

The **peripheral nervous system** includes nerves that run from the brain and spinal cord to the rest of the body. These nerves transmit sensations such as pain, temperature, and touch from the body to the spinal cord and brain (sensory nerves). Peripheral nerves also transmit impulses from the brain and spinal cord to the muscles (motor nerves). **Peripheral neuropathy** is the term used by physicians to describe disease of the peripheral nerves. Although peripheral neuropathy can afflict the sensory nerves as well as the motor nerves, the peripheral neuropathy experienced by myeloma patients is usually a sensory neuropathy resulting from nerve damage due to exposure to thalidomide, Velcade, or vincristine or directly from the myeloma itself. Patients with preexisting conditions that cause neuropathy are more commonly affected. Peripheral neuropathy is usually felt at first as a tingling and numbness in the hands and feet. Later symptoms can include burning sensations, shooting pain, throbbing, aching, and a feeling of "frostbite" or "walking on a bed of coals."

Peripheral neuropathy is a common, potentially severe side effect of treatment with thalidomide that may be irreversible. It generally occurs following chronic use of thalidomide over a period of months, but it sometimes can occur relatively quickly after short-term use. The symptoms sometimes improve after the thalidomide is discontinued. However, they may also resolve slowly or not at all. Velcade can also cause a sensory peripheral neuropathy that appears to be more common and more severe in patients who have previously been exposed to other drugs that can cause nerve damage such as thalidomide and vincristine. Peripheral neuropathy from Velcade tends to be resolved when Velcade is dose-reduced or discontinued in many patients.

The effects of neuropathy can be minimized by regular assessments by your physician (for example, at monthly intervals for the first 3 months of therapy and periodically thereafter) to detect early signs of neuropathy. You should inform your physician of any numbness, tingling, or pain in the hands and feet. If symptoms of drug-induced neuropathy develop, the drug should be discontinued or the dosage reduced immediately to limit further damage. Other medications known to be associated with neuropathy should be used with caution in patients receiving thalidomide and Velcade. In patients with established neuropathy, gabapentin (Neurontin) and amitriptyline (Elavil) may be of benefit.

62. I no longer seem interested in sexual intercourse. How can I avoid compromising my relationship with my partner?

The fatigue and pain associated with myeloma and the side effects of the treatment can often suppress sexual desire and your ability to enjoy sex. It is possible for many patients with myeloma to continue to have sexual intercourse as long as their pain, anemia, and other symptoms are treated. Some treatments, such as thalidomide, may have an effect on the ability to have sexual intercourse. For men, the use of medications for treatment of erectile dysfunction may be helpful. It is therefore important to discuss any physical barriers to sex with your physician as well as with your partner.

Maintaining communication with your partner will allow you to address any frustrations that may arise. Consider seeking expert help, such as sexual therapy counselors, when necessary.

63. I have had difficulty sleeping since beginning on treatment for myeloma. What can I do?

Sleeping difficulty is common in patients with cancer. Anxiety and depression associated with the diagnosis, pain associated with bony lesions, and nausea and peripheral neuropathy associated with medication can all contribute to this problem. Patients taking high doses of corticosteroids are particularly prone to sleep disturbance, as these drugs alter the natural sleep/wake rhythms of your body.

When addressing your sleeping difficulty, it is first important to deal with any of the causes just mentioned that can be prevented or reversed. Several simple measures may help you avoid the need for medications to help you sleep:

- Try to go to bed at a regular time each night.
- Avoid sleeping during the day, even though you feel fatigued. This often disturbs your normal sleep pattern, leading to wakefulness at night.
- Avoid stimulants such as coffee after dinner.
- Try relaxation techniques and yoga.

If simple measures fail, ask your physician to prescribe a medication to help you sleep. It may take a trial of several different medications before you find one that suits you best. In some cases, medication targeting daytime anxiety may also be necessary.

64. What is home care?

Home care is a term used to mean any care service for your myeloma that is provided at home rather than in the hospital or outpatient clinic. Usually home care involves home visits by a skilled professional (most commonly a nurse, but it can be a physical therapist, occupational therapist, and so on) and requires a physician's order. As is the case for hospital care, the home care agency used and the number of treatments/visits allowed may be dictated by your insurance provider. Thus, when home care is being planned, it is important that your medical team understand any requirements or restrictions imposed by your insurance plan.

PART FIVE

Stem Cell Transplantation

What is a stem cell, and how can it help in treatment of my myeloma?

Why are stem cell transplants performed for myeloma?

What is the difference between a bone marrow transplant and a stem cell transplant?

More ...

65. What is a stem cell, and how can it help in treatment of my myeloma?

A stem cell is any cell in the body that is capable of renewing itself when it divides to produce progeny (or daughter) cells. Stem cells reside in all tissues of the body that undergo cell division. These cells usually make up only a tiny fraction of all the cells in that organ or system, but they are capable of generating other cells in that organ when they undergo cell division. The type of stem cell that is commonly referred to when cancer physicians and patients talk about "stem cell transplants" is the bone marrow or hematopoietic (literally meaning "blood forming") stem cell.

66. Why are stem cell transplants performed for myeloma?

The most common reason for performing stem cell transplants in cancer therapy is to enable the administration of higher doses of chemotherapy and/or radiation than is possible without the stem cell transplant. The normal bone marrow is very sensitive to chemotherapy and radiation—and it is this vulnerability of the bone marrow that normally limits how much chemotherapy or extensive radiation can be given to treat the cancer. There are some cancers (including myeloma) that may benefit from higher doses of chemotherapy and/or radiation than can normally be given. In this situation an accompanying stem cell transplant may be the only way to deliver the required higher doses of treatment to the patient. It has been demonstrated that the high-dose chemotherapy enabled by a stem cell transplant increases the complete response rate in myeloma, compared to those patients who receive conventional doses of chemotherapy and no stem cell transplant. It may also improve survival in patients with myeloma. In addition to this benefit, certain types of stem cell transplants (namely allogeneic stem cell transplants) enable the delivery of a powerful form of immune therapy against some cancers, including myeloma (see Question 68).

67. What is the difference between a bone marrow transplant and a stem cell transplant?

When these types of transplants were first performed, the stem cells were obtained directly from the bone marrow (usually from the hip bones), using a needle, with the patient under general anesthetic. Therefore, the procedure was called a **bone marrow transplant**. However, in the last 10 to 15 years, the required cells have increasingly been obtained from the peripheral blood. When the peripheral blood is the source of the stem cells, the procedure is called a **peripheral blood stem cell transplant**. In order to collect the stem cells from the peripheral blood, the cells, which normally reside in the bone marrow, are induced to temporarily migrate to the peripheral blood through the use of growth factor drugs (such as Neupogen), with or without some chemotherapy (this is called stem cell **mobilization**). The cells can then be collected relatively easily from the blood through a procedure called leukapheresis. Leukepheresis involves the passing of your blood through a machine which "skims" off some of the white blood cells, without using general anesthetic.

Peripheral blood stem cell collection has some additional advantages over the collection of stem cells from the marrow directly. Usually a larger number of stem

Bone marrow transplant

aspiration of bone marrow fluid followed by infusion of the marrow into a patient. The source of the marrow can be the patient or a healthy individual.

Peripheral blood stem cell transplant

a procedure like bone marrow transplantation that uses stem cells derived from blood rather than marrow.

Mobilization (of stem cells)

the process whereby stem cells that normally reside in the bone marrow are induced to migrate into the blood temporarily, where they circulate and can be collected (harvested) for a subsequent transplant.

cells can be collected in this way, and the loss of red blood cells and other blood components is minimal compared to a bone marrow collection. In principle, the two types of transplant (bone marrow and peripheral blood) are otherwise very similar and are generally used for the same purpose. Sometimes the term "bone marrow transplant" is used loosely to cover either procedure.

Whereas peripheral blood stem cells have almost completely replaced bone marrow for autologous transplantation, bone marrow is still used in many centers for allogeneic transplantation (see Question 68).

68. What are the important differences between autologous and allogeneic transplantation?

Both autologous and allogeneic stem cell transplants are performed for patients with myeloma. For **autologous** stem cell transplantation, the patient's *own* stem cells are collected, usually after the patient has responded to several cycles of treatment. For **allogeneic** transplants, the stem cells collected are from a donor. Usually this is a brother or sister who is a match for the patient, or it may be a matched unrelated donor.

Both types of stem cell transplant enable the use of higher doses of chemotherapy or radiation than would otherwise be possible. However, allogeneic transplants also provide a form of **immune therapy** against myeloma that is not provided by autologous transplants. This is because when stem cells are collected, immune cells (called T-lymphocytes or T-cells) are included in the collection. Because the donor and the patient are *not* genetically identical, the donor's

T-lymphocytes use the genetic differences between the donor and patient to attack the patient's myeloma cells.

The cells obtained from the donor for an allogeneic transplant are derived from a normal individual, so they are practically guaranteed to be free of tumor contamination. On the other hand, cells collected from the patient for autologous transplant may possibly be contaminated with myeloma cells. It is unclear whether this possible contamination is of practical significance following autologous transplantation. Methods designed to purge the stem cell collection of contaminating myeloma cells have not been shown to improve the outcome in autologous transplantation.

Overall, the risk of myeloma relapse following allogeneic transplantation is lower than that following autologous transplantation. Also, there are reports of long-term survival among patients who have had allogeneic transplants. These patients may be cured of their myeloma. Long-term survival without eventual relapse is very rare following autologous transplantation alone. However, the risk of treatment-related complications, which may be severe enough to cause death, is significantly higher following allogeneic transplantation. The risk of these complications is higher in older patients and those using unrelated donors. Presently, allogeneic transplantation is not an appropriate treatment strategy for all patients with myeloma, but it may be useful to certain patients (such as younger patients and those with fully matched related donors).

One approach that is being assessed in the treatment of myeloma is to perform: an autologous transplant

Immune therapy
use of the immune system of the body to fight disease.

Stem Cell Transplantation

followed by an allogeneic one. Here, the patient undergoes high-dose chemotherapy with an autologous stem cell transplant in order to substantially decrease the myeloma cells in their body. The patient then has a nonablative (mini) allogeneic transplant (see Question 72), in order to offer a chance of long-term eradication of his or her myeloma. In such tandem transplants, the autologous transplant is designed to minimize the number of remaining myeloma cells that the allogeneic transplant has to deal with. Early reports regarding this approach appear promising, but the results of larger clinical trials with longer patient follow-up are still being awaited.

69. How is it decided which type of stem cell transplant is appropriate for me?

Generally speaking, almost all patients with advanced (Stage II or III) myeloma who are not either very elderly (more than 75 years old) or very debilitated by either their disease or coexisting medical conditions are potential candidates for autologous transplantation and may benefit from a consult with a stem cell transplant specialist. If you are a potential candidate for a stem cell transplant, your oncologist will refer you to a stem cell transplant specialist (if he or she is not such a specialist). The transplant specialist may be in the same treatment center, in a different treatment center, or even in a different city from your oncologist. Usually the stem cell transplant specialist will be one who your oncologist has a comfortable working relationship with and who works with your health insurance plan. After assessing your history, physical examination and medical records, the transplant specialist will confer with your oncologist to determine whether a stem cell transplant is appropriate for you.

The available stem cell transplant options include a single autologous transplant alone, double autologous transplantation, autologous followed by a mini-allogeneic transplant, or (rarely) allogeneic transplantation alone. In choosing among these approaches, your physicians will be influenced by your age, your general health, your social circumstances and support structure, the aggressiveness of your myeloma, the response obtained to standard-dose initial therapy for your myeloma, the availability and type of donor, your expectations from your treatment (for example, maximizing the chance of a cure versus minimizing side effects), and your tolerance of the risks of the proposed therapy. Ideally, the final choice will be made jointly by the physicians and you, once you are sufficiently informed regarding the issues involved. Some approaches may be available only within the context of a clinical trial, and your willingness to participate in the trial may determine the choice of therapy.

70. Are two autologous transplants better than one?

Because autologous stem cell transplants are generally very well tolerated by myeloma patients, some researchers have assessed the potential benefits of two consecutive autologous transplants for the treatment of myeloma. The objective of this approach is to attempt to increase the number of patients who achieve a complete remission and improve the overall outcome of myeloma patients. In order to perform a double autologous transplant, an attempt is made to collect enough stem cells prior to the first transplant to be sufficient for both of the transplants.

The role of such double transplants remains unclear at present. A large clinical trial in France has demonstrated a benefit to the double transplant over a single transplant in some groups of myeloma patients. Specifically, patients who do not achieve at least a partial response to their pretransplant treatment and patients who fail to achieve a complete remission after the first autologous transplant may benefit from a second autologous transplant. However, these results await confirmation.

71. I have had one previous autologous transplant. My myeloma has now relapsed. Is there any value in having a second transplant now?

Depending upon the type of response you had to your first autologous transplant and how long it took for your disease to relapse, you may benefit from a second such procedure. This works best if enough stem cells were originally collected to perform two transplants and your physician has stored enough cells for a second transplant. If there are no stored cells, or not enough of them, your physician will have to attempt to collect more cells through mobilization (see Question 67), which can be difficult after a previous transplant. The patients most likely to benefit from a second transplant are those who tolerated their first transplant well and had a relatively prolonged response to it. A second autologous transplant does not provide a cure but can provide months to a year or so without the need for further therapy. Other alternatives to consider at this stage are thalidomide, Velcade, chemotherapy, and, for selected patients, an allogeneic transplant.

72. What is a nonablative (mini) allogeneic transplant?

Although allogeneic transplantation has several potential advantages over autologous transplantation alone, it has in the past been associated with a relatively high risk of treatment-related complications and treatment-related death. Traditionally, an allogeneic transplant is performed using very high doses of chemotherapy and radiation designed to ablate, or destroy, the patient's bone marrow and immune system before they are regenerated using stem cells from the donor. Patients with myeloma are usually somewhat older than patients receiving stem cell transplants for other cancers, and their immune system is already suppressed by their myeloma. As a result, these patients have difficulty in tolerating such ablative preparative regimens for their allogeneic transplant.

More recently, a newer approach to allogeneic stem cell transplants has been evaluated that utilizes much lower doses of chemotherapy and/or radiation to prepare myeloma patients for their transplant. This approach is called nonablative allogeneic transplantation (also known as nonmyeloablative, reduced-intensity, or mini transplantation). To prepare for such transplants, the physicians do not eliminate the patient's bone marrow but provide just enough temporary suppression of the immune system to allow the donor's cells to establish themselves in the patient's body after their infusion. The donor's immune cells

(T-lymphocytes) then mount an immune attack that slowly eradicates any remaining stem cells and immune cells left over from the patient. Although this approach does not remove all the risks associated with allogeneic transplantation (see Question 73), the data acquired so far suggest that the risk of treatment-related complications and death in the early period after the transplant seems substantially lower than that seen following traditional (ablative) transplants performed for myeloma.

This nonablative approach may enable patients who would not previously have been candidates for allogeneic transplantation to have access to this form of therapy. In patients who have a donor and are otherwise suitable candidates, nonablative allogeneic transplantation is often performed after a patient has recovered from an autologous transplant (tandem autologous-allogeneic transplantation; see Question 68). Presently, this approach is being compared to two consecutive autologous transplants followed by maintenance thalidomide in a large clinical trial throughout the United States in order to determine which approach produces the best outcomes.

73. What complications can occur following stem cell transplants?

Both autologous and allogeneic stem cell transplants have become safer over the last few years. However, a risk of complication exists with either procedure that any potential candidate for this therapy must be fully aware of.

Autologous stem cell transplants are now considered very safe procedures. The risk of death from this procedure is now in the 1 to 3% range in most large transplant centers. The procedure appears to be well tolerated in otherwise healthy patients who are up to 70 to 75 years old. The potential risks include bacterial infections during the period when the white blood count is very low from the chemotherapy. Because a central venous catheter is present, it can sometimes become infected during this time. Some patients develop a sore mouth and throat and stomach cramps and diarrhea from damage to the lining of the mouth and the rest of gut by the high-dose chemotherapy administered. These symptoms are usually temporary and can be controlled with painkillers and other medications. Occasionally patients develop liver and kidney dysfunction during the procedure. This is usually mild and temporary.

Allogeneic transplants have a higher overall risk of treatment-related complications than autologous transplants, Patients having an allogeneic transplant can have all the potential complications described for autologous transplants. However, the risk of complications caused by the high-dose chemotherapy given immediately prior to the transplant is reduced in patients who have a nonablative allogeneic transplant (see Question 72).

In addition to the risks described for autologous transplants, patients who undergo an allogeneic transplant have risks of infections and immune complications that are more specific to this type of transplant. After an allogeneic transplant, the patient has a severely suppressed immune system for a much longer period than following an autologous transplant. This is associated with a risk of developing unusual infections. To prevent these, it is usually necessary to take anti-infection medications for several months after the transplant. There is also a risk that the immune cells (T-lymphocytes) that are transplanted from the donor will attack some normal organs in the body (in addition to the myeloma cells). This phenomenon is referred to as **graft-versus-host-disease (GVHD)** and is a risk associated only with allogeneic (not autologous) transplants. See Question 74 for a further discussion of GVHD.

Graft-versus-host disease (GVHD)

a complication of allogeneic stem cell transplantation that results from an immune attack against the normal organs of the patient.

Because allogeneic transplants involve a transfer of cells from donor to patient, there is a possibility of transplant rejection if the donor's immune system is not adequately suppressed before the transplant. If the patient has had an ablative transplant (see Question 72), this rejection can result in a prolonged period with very low blood counts and is potentially fatal. It is usually treated by repeating the transplant using stronger immune-suppression medications before the procedure. When transplant rejection occurs following a nonablative transplant, the patient's own blood cells usually recover, making the complication less serious in the short term. However, another transplant is usually required in order to treat the patient's myeloma.

Because of these additional complications, the risk of death is significantly higher following allogeneic transplants than following autologous ones. The exact risk is difficult to determine and depends upon your age, the type of donor used (matched brother or sister versus unrelated donor), the presence of other unrelated health problems, nonablative versus ablative transplant, and so on. Otherwise healthy patients in their

50s or 60s undergoing a nonablative transplant from a matched sibling will have at least a 15% chance of dying from complications of the treatment.

74. What is graft–versus–host disease?

Graft-versus-host disease (GVHD) is a condition that can happen after an allogeneic stem cell transplant but not after an autologous one. The incoming immune cells from the donor after an allogeneic stem cell transplant are genetically distinct from the patient's cells. This difference is used by the donor immune cells to attack and possibly eradicate the patient's myeloma. However, if this reaction is vigorous, the immune cells can also attack normal organs in the patient's body, and this is known as GVHD.

When GVHD occurs in the first 3 months after the transplant (acute GVHD), it can involve the skin, the gut, and the liver, causing a rash, diarrhea, and abnormal liver function tests, respectively. Later in the course of the transplant, symptoms can be more chronic, and several other organs may be affected, including the mouth, eyes, joints, and lungs in addition to the organs just mentioned (chronic GVHD). To prevent GVHD, patients take medications for several months after the transplant. When GVHD occurs following the transplant, it is usually mild to moderate and can be controlled by a change of medications. Mild GVHD can be beneficial, as it is associated with a lowering of the risk of relapse of the myeloma. However, a minority of patients develop more severe GVHD, which can be fatal if it does not respond adequately to treatment. Usually the risk of severe GVHD is related to the age of the patient and the level of matching between the patient and donor.

75. What is a donor leukocyte infusion?

Although allogeneic transplantation can potentially eradicate myeloma, some patients will relapse even after this procedure. When a relapse occurs following an allogeneic transplant, it can often be treated with a simple infusion of additional immune cells from the donor, without any further chemotherapy or immune-suppression treatments. This is called a **donor lymphocyte (or leukocyte) infusion (DLI)**. A DLI can sometimes produce a complete remission of the relapsed myeloma. However, it can take several weeks to be effective, and therefore this approach works best in early relapse when the patient's myeloma is not at risk of rapidly becoming overwhelming. Also, a DLI does not work in all cases, and it carries with it a risk of inducing GVHD (see Question 74). This risk can be lowered by giving a small dose of cells to start with. Larger doses of cells are then given later if no response occurs following the lower dose (this is known as dose escalation).

Donor lymphocyte infusion (DLI)

administration of additional donor cells to a patient some time after an allogeneic transplant. Usually no additional preparative treatment is administered prior to the infusion of these cells.

76. How does an allogeneic transplant from a related donor differ from one from an unrelated donor?

Every full sibling (brother or sister from the same two parents) has an approximately 25% chance of being a perfect match for the patient for the purpose of a stem cell transplant. Such **matched sibling donors** (also known as HLA-identical sibling donors) have been the most commonly used donors for allogeneic stem cell transplantation for myeloma. However, because of

Matched sibling donors

A transplant donor who is a full brother or sister who matches the patient for tissue type.

the small average size of a family in most Western countries, most patients will not have a matched sibling donor available. For such patients, a **matched unrelated donor (MUD)** can potentially be used. Matched unrelated donors are found through a search of the available registries of volunteer donors. The largest such registry is the National Marrow Donor Program (NMDP, *www.marrow.org*), which has in excess of five million registered donors. The chances of finding an MUD are relatively high, depending upon the patient's ethnicity (> 80% for Caucasians, lower for African-Americans).

Unrelated donor transplants have some disadvantages compared to related donor transplants:

- Finding an unrelated donor takes much longer than finding a matched sibling donor if one is present. Finding such a donor requires detailed testing of donor specimens, and it can take 4 to 6 months from starting a search to being able to do the transplant.
- Transplants from unrelated donors have higher rates of GVHD and graft rejection than transplants from matched sibling donors.

Traditionally, unrelated donor transplants have had a lower success rate than transplants from matched siblings. However, recent advances in techniques for matching patient to donor have led to improvements in outcomes following unrelated donor transplants.

JWH: The first advice I received was to have the autologous transplant followed by the mini allogeneic transplant. While considering that advice, I obtained a second opinion from a noted myeloma doctor who told me not to get a

Matched unrelated donor (MUD)

an unrelated transplant donor who is matched with the patient for tissue type.

Stem Cell Transplantation

transplant at all. In the meantime, I had my one sister tested for compatibility and found out that she was an HLA match. I was then faced with the decision of whether to undergo the transplants, especially in the face of conflicting recommendations by two reputable physicians. After much consideration and prayer, I decided to go through with them. I would suggest that if you have siblings, and you are at least considering a transplant, you have them tested to see if they are a match so you can make a fully informed decision.

77. I don't have a sibling donor. Should my friend/neighbor/cousin get tested?

The chances of unrelated individuals being a match for a patient they know are almost infinitesimally small. Thus, the cost of testing such individuals as potential donors for you is not worth it. On the other hand, any individual can get tested as a potential donor by volunteering to be listed on the NMDP's registry of donors. Volunteering in this way may allow him or her to help another individual who is in need of a transplant.

The chances of a cousin or other distant relative being a match are also very small, and thus typing of all available relatives is not recommended. The chance that a first-degree relative other than a sibling (for example, a parent or child) being a match is typically 2 to 3% for each such relative. If no other suitable donor can be found, such first-degree relatives can be tested.

78. What is a cord-blood transplant?

The blood drained from the placenta through the umbilical cord contains hematopoietic stem cells and can be used for an allogeneic transplant. Several "banks" of such cord-blood units exist, and they can be searched for a potential unit to use for an allogeneic transplant. However, because the units contain only a relatively small number of stem cells, they are more useful for transplants in children than in adults with myeloma.

PART SIX

If Treatment Fails

How do I decide whether active treatment is
no longer worthwhile?

What is comfort care?

If I stop active anticancer therapy, what other
options are available?

More . . .

79. How do I decide whether active treatment is no longer worthwhile?

The choice to stop active treatment for your myeloma is an intensely personal and individual one. As a general rule, most patients consider stopping active anticancer treatment when the prospect of obtaining a response that produces a meaningful prolongation of life or improvement in symptoms is outweighed by the likelihood of having significant side effects from the therapy, which will likely worsen their quality of life. However, the actual point at which such a decision is appropriate for you will vary depending upon your objectives, your philosophy, the opinion of relatives and friends you trust, the advice of your physician, and so on. Patients who are competent to make the decision must make it for themselves. Prior discussion of this issue with close relatives and friends before the question becomes urgent will help clarify your own feelings and resolve any conflicts that may exist.

80. What is comfort care?

When deciding against further active anticancer treatment, the patient and close family and friends may elect to have comfort care. This allows the treating physician to concentrate on measures designed to ensure the patient's comfort and freedom from distress rather than to prolong life. Tests and medications are minimized except those that have a clearly beneficial impact on the patient's immediate quality of life. Active treatment of the myeloma—for example, with chemotherapy—is not typically used in the comfort care mode, as such therapy is unlikely to cause regression of the myeloma and is very likely to produce side effects that will significantly impair the patient's quality of life.

81. If I stop active anticancer therapy, what other options are available?

After discontinuation of active anticancer therapies, you can continue to take advantage of the many ancillary therapies that are focused on improving your quality of life. These include medications to relieve pain, nausea, diarrhea, anxiety, and depression. Antibiotics can also be used to treat infections that cause symptoms. The objective is to relieve any distressing symptoms you may have as completely as possible so that you can spend quality time with your loved ones.

82. What is hospice, and how can it help?

Hospice is a specialized form of end-of-life care. Hospice services usually involve a multidisciplinary team comprising trained individuals who are focused upon making life for the terminally ill patient as symptom-free and productive as possible. The team includes physicians, nurses, social workers, spiritual counselors, and others who are assembled to address the medical, emotional, and practical needs of the patient who is terminally ill.

Patients who qualify for hospice care generally have an anticipated life expectancy of 6 months or less and have elected to emphasize quality of life rather than life prolongation. Aggressive anticancer therapy aimed at prolonging life or achieving a cure is usually not compatible with hospice care. However, some types of anticancer therapy, such as chemotherapy and radiation therapy, may be allowed if they are determined to be the best way to relieve symptoms.

Hospice care is usually provided in the patient's home, where the hospice team visits regularly and assists in

If Treatment Fails

the care provided by your family. However, hospice services can also be provided on an inpatient basis in a hospital or skilled nursing facility. Your oncologist or social worker can usually direct you to an appropriate hospice facility for your needs.

83. What is a DNR order?

DNR stands for "do not resuscitate." A **DNR order** is an order written in the patient's chart in accordance with his or her wishes. It states that if the patient either stops breathing or his or her heart stops, acute resuscitative measures designed to keep the patient alive will *not* be started. Why would a patient decide this? When a patient has a terminal condition such as a cancer that cannot be cured, and has a relatively short life expectancy, the stopping of the heart or the cessation of breathing is a natural event that signals the end of life. It is the natural end result of the progression of the patient's cancer. "Heroic" measures designed to bring the patient back to life are almost always unsuccessful in this instance. If such measures are started, they usually result in an agonizing period during which the patient may be subjected to painful and undignified procedures (such as chest compression and mouth-to-mouth resuscitation, insertion of venous and arterial catheters, and artificial ventilation on a machine), which are almost always futile in bringing the patient back for any meaningful length of time. The patient's next of kin is often then faced with a difficult decision to turn off life-support measures so that the patient can die.

Most patients with terminal cancer wish to avoid this situation and instead choose to pass away in a digni-

DNR order

"do not resuscitate" is a formal order written in a patient's medical chart indicating that at the patient's or family's request, acute measures to keep the patient alive will not be started.

fied and peaceful way in the company of their loved ones. The DNR order is a way of allowing this to happen. It states that the nurses looking after the patient will not "call a code" (summon the crash team to resuscitate the patient) in the event that the patient's heart or breathing stop. However, the choice of a DNR order versus full resuscitative measures must be made by each patient individually.

Ideally, the issue of a DNR order should be discussed among the patient, his or her loved ones, and the treating physician before the patient's condition has seriously deteriorated, even though the issue may be uncomfortable for all involved. This will allow the patient and his or her family and friends to discuss the issue in a calm and objective way and will give them an opportunity to comprehend the issues and have their questions answered.

84. What is an advance directive?

An advance directive is a legal agreement that clarifies your wishes for your future medical care in the event that you become incapacitated. Two major types of advance directive are commonly used by cancer patients. A **living will** is a document specifying your treatment wishes in the event you are unable to decide these questions in the future. In such a will you can specify a DNR order, other preferences regarding life-support machines such as ventilators and dialysis machines, nutrition and hydration, and your preferences regarding organ and tissue donation. A **medical power of attorney** names an individual who will make health care decisions for you in the event that you are unable to make them for yourself. This individual

Living will

a document specifying an individual's treatment wishes in the event that he or she is unable to decide these questions.

Medical power of attorney

a document that designates an individual who will make healthcare decisions on behalf of someone who is unable to do this for himself.

should normally be close to you and should be able to make decisions based upon a knowledge of what you would have wished under the circumstances.

Advance directives can be made using an attorney or simply by using forms provided by the hospital you are treated at or downloaded from the Internet. One source is *www.partnershipforcaring.org*.

85. If my disease becomes fatal, how can I prepare for my death?

Despite the emotional distress for you and your family that can be associated with the realization that death may be imminent, it may be necessary to take several actions to prepare for your death. Create advance directives if these are not already in place. This will prevent decisions being made that you would not have supported.

It is important to address your financial affairs, including a will. This will ensure that your family and loved ones do not face additional burdens after your death. It is essential to communicate with loved ones and not to avoid dealing with the emotional aspects. Attending to your spiritual needs, whether or not you are religious, will also help.

Someone who specializes in the needs of terminally ill patients may provide invaluable assistance. Seeking hospice care can help address a number of these issues.

PART SEVEN

Advocacy and Support

Does myeloma run in families? Are my relatives at risk?

Should I receive immunoglobulin therapy?

Can I have a flu shot?

More . . .

86. Does myeloma run in families? Are my relatives at risk?

The exact cause of myeloma is unknown. Exposure to radiation may contribute to the disease, and it is more common among African-Americans than people of other races. However, myeloma is not typically an inherited disease, and family members of myeloma patients are considered to be at only slightly greater risk. Very rarely, clusters of myeloma cases have been described in some families. The existence of such a cluster is not proof that the myeloma was inherited. Instead, common exposure to an environmental agent may have contributed. Also, no infectious agent has been reliably identified as a cause of myeloma. Thus, myeloma cannot be transmitted to family members through contact.

87. Should I receive immunoglobulin therapy?

Advanced stage myeloma can be associated with a severe reduction on the levels of normal blood immunoglobulin proteins. This can predispose one to recurrent bacterial infections. The levels of the normal immunoglobulins often recover when the myeloma goes into remission after treatment. However, many patients may be left with very low levels of normal immunoglobulin. In patients who develop recurrent bacterial infections in the presence of severely depressed levels of normal immunoglobulin that are likely to be chronic, infusions of intravenous immunoglobulin (IVIG) can sometimes be useful. However, the treatment is very expensive and results in exposure to proteins from other individuals (although these proteins are treated to prevent transmission of blood-borne infections).

88. Can I have a flu shot?

Flu vaccinations are recommended for myeloma patients, as the consequences of flu can be serious for these patients. Myeloma itself is not a reason to avoid the flu vaccination.

89. What is a pneumonia vaccine, and do I need it?

Pneumonia vaccine (sometimes known as Pneumovax) protects against pneumonia and blood infections caused by a bacterium called pneumococcus. This is a serious and potentially life-threatening infection that is more common in patients with a compromised immune system, such as myeloma patients. Such a vaccination may be a good idea if your physician believes it is called for. A repeat vaccination is usually recommended every five years.

90. Is work possible while undergoing treatment?

Your ability to continue to work will depend upon the effects that the myeloma has already had on your body and the intensity of your treatment and on any side effects you may experience. Many patients find that they can continue to work during at least part of their therapies. However, you may need to reduce your work hours or stop work completely for a period if you are physically disabled or significantly fatigued by your treatments or by the myeloma.

If you have to take sick leave, it is important to consult with the human resources professional or social worker at your place of work to ensure that you do not lose

Advocacy and Support

health benefits due to prolonged periods off work. If you are unable to work for long periods, you may need to seek disability benefits.

91. Can I exercise?

Exercise remains important in myeloma patients, including those undergoing treatment. Its potential benefits include maintaining your physical conditioning, increasing strength and energy, elevating your mood, and improving sleep. These factors in turn help you cope better with the rigors of your disease and its therapy.

Aerobic exercise such as brisk walking for 20 to 30 minutes three to five times a week, using a stationary exercise bicycle, and swimming are likely to be the most beneficial.

Weight-bearing exercise, and exercise that subjects you to potential physical injury such as mountain bicycling, contact sports, and so on can be much more risky for patients with myeloma than for those with some other cancers. This is because the weakening of the bone associated with lytic lesions or generalized osteoporosis caused by the myeloma can enormously increase the risk of fractures from those activities. Thus, before embarking on any such exercise, it is important to consult with your physician, who can assess the potential for such fractures in your case with x-rays and other imaging tests.

JWH: When I was diagnosed, I was in good health. I ran five or more times a week, lifted weights, and commonly participated in other activities. It was difficult for me to imagine my days without exercise. I asked my doctor about continuing to run, and he was very hesitant because I had weakened bones and several lesions that were identified by a bone scan. Still, he told me I could walk, and gave me permission to begin running again fairly quickly. I have been able to exercise throughout my treatment. There have been weeks when I couldn't exercise because of weakness, but I have always returned to routine exercise, outside, in the fresh air, with friends. I have found it invigorating and helpful, both physically and psychologically. Additionally, if you are going to have a transplant, the doctors will check the condition of your lungs and heart to make sure you can endure the high-dose chemotherapy. The better the shape you're in, the easier it will be to tolerate this treatment.

I would strongly suggest that you continue to exercise throughout your treatment whenever you are able. Even if you're in the hospital, walk around as much as you can. Realize that this is a battle, and part of the physical battle will be determined by what kind of shape your body is in during the fight. Much of the battle is psychological as well, and your state of mind will be helped beyond measure by a good exercise program.

92. Do I need to change my diet?

Although patients often hear from friends and family members that certain unusual diets will dramatically affect their disease and survival, there is in fact no strong evidence that a particular type of diet has any major beneficial influence upon the outcome of myeloma, and some diets, such as those high in folic acid or antioxidants, have the potential of interfering with treatments for your myeloma.

However, it is still important to pay some attention to your diet. You can follow general guidelines for healthy eating in cancer patients, such as the guidelines provided by the American Cancer Society. They include the following: eat five or more servings of a variety of vegetables and fruits each day; choose whole grains in preference to processed (refined) grains and sugars; limit consumption of red meats, especially those high in fat and processed; and choose foods that help maintain a healthful weight. (See the American Cancer Society web site for details: *www.cancer.org.*)

Supplementing your diet with large quantities of vitamins or herbal supplements has not been proven to improve outcomes in myeloma and may in some cases be harmful or interfere with therapy.

There are nutritionists who specialize in assisting cancer patients. Although the evidence is usually anecdotal, many patients believe that consulting with such nutritionists is beneficial. If you decide to consult with a nutritionist, be sure to keep your physician informed of what you are doing to ensure that your actions are not counterproductive to your primary treatment.

JWH: As I stated earlier, count me as one who thinks that nutrition can make a difference in your treatment. I don't want get too deeply into a discussion of what is proven or not by medical standards. There is much to be said on both sides of that debate. But as one patient to another, I highly recommend that you consult with a nutritionist to discuss your options for dietary changes and supplements. There are things that you can do, many of them very simple, that may help in your treatment or recovery. In considering a nutritionist's suggestions, you may conclude that the evidence in support of nutrition is, in fact, anecdotal. But you may still want to try them, in the "it can't hurt" theory of treatment.

I think it is very fair to say that a healthy diet cannot hurt you. You'll have to decide for yourself whether to take supplements (I do) and what benefit they might have for you. You won't find much support for using supplements in the usual medical circles, because of the lack of evidence to substantiate their value. But frankly, I was at the stage (Stage IIIB) where anecdotal evidence was good enough for me, if there wasn't much risk of harm.

Decide for yourself. Do the research. Find out what evidence there is, and do what you think is best. But do keep your oncologist informed of all that you are doing, so you don't accidentally settle on something that might be counterproductive.

93. I have lost a lot of weight during treatment, and I have no appetite. What can I do?

Patients who have specific nutritional problems, such as weight loss, resulting from their myeloma or its therapy will, of course, need special diets (for example, calorie-enriched, high-protein diets) to reverse the problem. Usually a consult with a nutritionist is a good idea. You may also need to control your nausea, high blood calcium, and other medical problems. Sometimes you may require treatments such as megestrol acetate (Megace), which is a hormonal treatment that can help stimulate appetite in cancer patients. In patients who are unable to take oral nutrition for physical reasons, such as difficulty swallowing, inflammation of the mouth or esophagus from treatment or infection, and so on, feeding via a tube that is passed from nose to stomach may be temporarily necessary. In some patients who have failed to stabilize their weight through other types of nutrition, intravenous (parenteral) nutrition may be necessary for a short period. However, such nutrition often requires placement of an indwelling venous catheter (a catheter that is left in place) and can increase the patient's susceptibility to infection.

94. How do I tell my friends and relatives about my diagnosis?

Talking to others about your diagnosis/prognosis and the progress of your treatment is not easy for many people. Having a cancer such as myeloma may change your relationship with people you know. Often this is for the better, but sometimes it is for the worse. Do not try to keep your diagnosis a secret. It is likely to increase any loneliness you may feel in coping with your disease. Of course, you first need to be ready to talk about your illness and your concerns. So if you are not quite ready, it is not unreasonable to inform your loved ones that you will talk when the time is right, while reassuring them that you appreciate their concern.

Some people you know may have trouble coping with your diagnosis. They may withdraw or call and visit less frequently. Often this is because they are not sure what to say or do not wish to be inappropriate. If the relationships are ones that you value, you may have to make the first move—to call and reassure them that you value the relationship and are willing to honestly discuss any fears they may have. If they fail to respond to your overtures, it is unlikely that the relationships will be worth pursuing. It is possible that some people you love will disappoint you. On the other hand, there will be many others who will impress you with their strength and determination to be by your side.

JWH: You are about to learn a lot of things about people you thought you knew well. Some of your closest friends will go quiet on you. Some people you barely know may begin visiting you and supporting you way beyond where people you've known for decades are willing to go.

One thing you may find annoying is that many people will now regard you as a "patient." Perhaps when you used to see people, they'd ask about your children, or your job, or a baseball team—whatever they thought of when they saw you. But now they'll ask you—probably every time they see you—"How are you doing?" or "How are your numbers?" since they'll soon learn that we typically monitor our condition with blood tests and "numbers." It becomes mind-numbing to have the same conversation over and over again all day long, and then again the next day. I began just saying, "I'm fine." They of course knew that I wasn't, but tended not to push it.

Additionally, you'll find that some people just seem willing to ask questions that they really shouldn't. Feel free to say that you would like to talk about something else, and that you'll keep them posted on any big developments.

95. Should I join a support group?

A **support group** consists of a group of patients with the same or similar types of cancer, usually led by a facilitator who can be a health professional or a patient leader. Some support groups bring together patients with different cancers who have undergone a particular type of treatment, such as bone marrow transplant or chemotherapy. The group may be very structured or very informal with a social emphasis. Most support groups provide a forum for you to interact with other

Support group

a group of patients with the same or similar disease offering the opportunity to share information and experience with others.

patients who may be in a situation similar to yours or who have undergone similar treatments, so that you can share and learn from each other's experiences. Attending a support group can also alleviate feelings of isolation that you or members of your family may feel when coping with your myeloma. They also provide education about your disease and available treatments and other resources. This is usually achieved through scheduled speakers with whom you can interact and by the provision of published literature and other educational resources.

Increasing numbers of online support groups also exist for those patients who are unable or unwilling to travel to support group meetings. It is important to remember that information obtained through a support group is not necessarily screened for accuracy and may be colored by the biases of the provider of the information. This is particularly true of online support groups. It is therefore important to discuss any knowledge you receive from support groups with your health professionals in order to gain their perspective.

If you want to participate in a support group, you can obtain information about local groups from your physician, nurse, or social worker. Lists of support group contacts by location are also maintained on the web sites of the International Myeloma Foundation (www.myeloma. org) and the Multiple Myeloma Research Foundation (*www.multiplemyeloma.org*). Other resources include the wellness community (*www.thewellnesscommunity.org*) and the Association of Cancer Online resources (*www. acor.org*).

JWH: The Association of Cancer Online Resources maintains a multiple myeloma e-mail distribution list. It allows people *to exchange many common—and uncommon—questions and answers about myeloma on a daily basis. I found it very helpful to subscribe to the e-mail list, especially when I was first diagnosed. I was scared, confused, and baffled by the terminology. You can ask anything there, and someone will help you. Many people have been members of that list for years and have seen virtually all the questions you might have. You might want to subscribe for a while to see if it is helpful to you (*http://listserv.acor.org/archives/myeloma.html*).*

96. How can I protect myself financially against the expenses of therapy and loss of work?

Your myeloma and its treatment may place significant financial burdens upon you and your family. It is important to review the healthcare benefits of your medical insurance plan carefully so you understand what is and is not covered. This may require contacting a health benefits officer in the human resources department where you work or contacting the help line of your health plan. It may be helpful to delegate financial and insurance related issues to a trusted family member or friend while you concentrate on the medical aspects of your treatment. A meeting with the financial counselor or social worker at the cancer center where you are being treated may also help. This individual may also identify other financial resources (such as money to assist with transportation to and from care appointments, provided by the Leukemia and Lymphoma Society, Cancer Care, and the American Cancer Society) that may help with your out-of-pocket expenses.

It is important to find out whether your health plan is very restrictive about the healthcare providers (doctors, home care nurses, hospitals, pharmacies, and so forth) you can use, or whether you can choose among a wider variety of providers. In some cases you may be able to access out-of-network providers by paying a higher co-payment. You can also ask your health plan's staff about whether a second opinion is covered and who you can go to for this, what authorization process must be followed before you can receive tests or treatments, whether there are restrictions on prescription drug coverage, and whether annual or lifetime caps on healthcare costs are present in your plan.

If you plan to be off work temporarily or permanently, make sure that your insurance coverage is not lost in the process. Once again, you may need professional help to avoid the possibility of loss of coverage, which can be devastating to your financial and physical well-being.

97. I have received bills from the hospital, and they don't seem correct. What should I do?

You may receive invoices or bills directly from the hospital where you are being treated. It is important to clarify with your health plan or a counselor who understands your plan as to whether the charges are in line with the co-payments you are responsible for under your plan. Mistakes in such invoices are common. Usually the insurance plan will send you an explanation of benefits (EOB), which should explain the charges, the amount the insurance will pay, and any portion you are responsible for.

It is important to keep records and documentation of all invoices and payments that you make. This will help if mistakes need to be clarified. It will also help you be able to claim any tax deductions for your medical expenses to which you may be entitled (discuss these with an accountant).

98. My insurance company is denying treatment that I feel I am entitled to. What should I do?

If you have a dispute with your insurance company concerning denial of a treatment or test that you feel should be covered, you may be able to resolve the issue by communicating with your health plan, as a simple error may be responsible. Other times, additional medical information from your physician's office is all that is required. If this does not work and you feel the insurance company is wrong, you may address the issue with the Department of Health, Insurance, or Managed Care of your state government. A mechanism usually exists for filing a grievance, and for third-party review of your case at that level. Failing all other alternatives, you can hire an attorney with expertise in health insurance matters.

99. I have no medical insurance. Are there resources for me?

If you have no medical insurance coverage at the time you develop myeloma, you may be faced with major financial burdens, and you may have to use your available assets to pay for medical care.

It is important to contact a financial counselor or social worker at the cancer center where you plan to receive treatment as soon as possible, so that you can discuss any available options and access them if you are eligible. Options include Medicaid, a government insurance program for patients with limited or no financial assets who meet citizenship criteria; Medicare, a federally run insurance program for those who either are over the age of 65, are legally blind, have been on social security disability for two consecutive years, or are on renal dialysis (*www.medicare.gov*); and Veterans Affairs (VA) benefits for those with qualifying military service, which can provide all necessary health care within the VA system to those who qualify.

Some larger cancer centers may provide low-cost or free treatment to patients who do not have adequate health insurance and who meet their specific criteria. This availability varies from region to region.

Sometimes it is possible to access health care by participating in a clinical trial where the treatment and tests are paid for by the sponsor of the study. If you are eligible for such a clinical trial, you need to discuss the financial issues with the treating team before you sign up for the study, as many clinical trials expect insurance to pay for tests and treatments they consider part of "routine" management and not directly related to the study medication. The National Cancer Institute (NCI, *www.cancer.gov*) provides free treatment to patients who are eligible and who participate in one of their internal clinical trials. However, the treatments are usually administered at the NCI Center in Bethesda, Maryland (near Washington, D.C.). If you or your physician feel you are eligible for one of the clinical trials offered at the NCI, you will usually have to pay for initial transportation to Washington, D.C., to see the physician who is conducting the trial. Once the NCI team determines that you are eligible and you elect to participate in the study, your trips to Washington will be paid for while you remain in the study.

100. Where can I obtain additional information? How can I get involved with organizations that provide help and advocacy for patients with myeloma and their families?

Many organizations can provide additional information and help. A list of such organizations and available web sites is listed at the end of this book. The International Myeloma Foundation (*www.myeloma. org*), the Multiple Myeloma Research Foundation (*www.multiplemyeloma.org*), and the Leukemia & Lymphoma Society (*www.leukemia-lymphoma.org*) may be particularly useful in this regard.

Myeloma Information and Resources

International Myeloma Foundation
www.myeloma.org
12650 Riverside Drive, Suite 206
North Hollywood, CA 91607-3421
phone: 800-452-2873 (U.S. and Canada)
818-487-7455 (elsewhere)
fax: 818-487-7454
e-mail: *The IMF@myeloma.org*

Leukemia & Lymphoma Society
www.leukemia-lymphoma.org
1311 Mamaroneck Avenue
White Plains, NY 10605
phone: 914-949-5213; toll-free: 800-955-4572
fax: 914-949-6691

Multiple Myeloma Research Foundation
www.multiplemyeloma.org
51 Locust Avenue, Suite 201
New Canaan, CT 06840
phone: 203-972-1250
e-mail: *info@themmrf.org*

Other Organizations of Interest

American Cancer Society (ACS)
www.cancer.org
1599 Clifton Road
Atlanta, GA 30329
phone: 800-ACS-2345

American Society of Hematology (ASH)

www.hematology.org
1900 M Street NW, Suite 200
Washington, DC 20036
phone: 202-776-0544
fax: 202-776-0545

American Society of Clinical Oncology (ASCO)

www.asco.org
1900 Duke Street, Suite 200
Alexandria, VA 22314
phone: 703-299-0150
fax: 703-299-1044
e-mail: *asco@asco.org*

Association of Cancer Online Resources

www.listserv.acor.org/archives/myeloma.html

National Cancer Institute (NCI)

www.cancer.gov
NCI Public Information Office
Building 31, Room 10A31
31 Center Drive, MSC 2580
Bethesda, MD 20892-2580
phone: 301-435-3848

Clinical Trials Information from NCI

www.nci.nih.gov/clinical_trials

List of NCI-Designated Cancer Centers and Contact Information

http://www3.cancer.gov/cancercenters/centerslist.html

Cancer Care, Inc.

www.cancercare.org
275 7th Avenue
New York, NY 10001
phone: 800-813-HOPE (4637)
212-712-8400 (admin)
212-712-8080 (services)
fax: 212-712-8495
e-mail: *info@cancercare.org*

American Society for Blood and Marrow Transplantation
www.asbmt.org
85 W Algonquin Road, Suite 550
Arlington Heights, IL 60005
phone: 847-427-0224
fax: 847-427-9656
e-mail: *mail@asbmt.org*

International Bone Marrow Transplant Registry (IBMTR)/
Autologous Blood & Marrow Transplant Registry (ABMTR)
www.ibmtr.org
Medical College of Wisconsin
8701 Watertown Plank Road
P.O. Box 26509
Milwaukee, WI 53226
phone: 414-456-8325
fax: 414-456-6530
e-mail: *ibmtr@mew.edu*

National Marrow Donor Program
www.marrow.org
3001 Broadway Street Northeast, Suite 500
Minneapolis, MN 55413-1753
phone: 800-MARROW2 (800-627-7692)
Office of Patient Advocacy (OPA): 888-999-6743

Blood & Marrow Transplant Information Network
www.bmtinfonet.org
2900 Skokie Valley Road, Suite B
Highland Park, IL 60035
phone: 847-433-3313; toll-free: 888-597-7674
fax: 847-433-4599
e-mail: *help@bmtinfonet.org*

Wellness Community
www.thewellnesscommunity.org
919 18th Street NW, Suite 54
Washington, DC 20006
phone: 202-659-9709; toll-free: 888-793-WELL
fax: 202-659-9301

Well Spouse Foundation

www.wellspouse.org
63 West Main Street, Suite H
Freehold, NJ 07728
phone: 800-838-0879

Neuropathy Association

www.neuropathy.org
60 E 42nd Street, Suite 942
New York, NY 10165-0999
phone: 212-692-0662

National Pain Foundation (NPF)

www.painconnection.org
P.O. Box 102606
Denver, CO 80250-2605

Patient Advocate Foundation

www.patientadvocate.org
700 Thimble Shoals Blvd, Suite 200
Newport News, VA 23606
phone: 800-532-5274

Centers for Medicare and Medicaid Services (CMS)

www.cms.hhs.gov

Veterans Health Administration

www1.va.gov/health_benefits
810 Vermont Avenue NW
Washington, DC 20420
phone: 202-273-5400; toll-free: 877-222-8387

Social Security Administration

www.ssa.gov

Glossary

Advance directive: A legal document that indicates a patient's wishes with respect to his or her treatment and other matters if the patient becomes incapacitated and unable to make decisions. Such a document can also name another individual who can make decisions for the patient in this event. See also *durable power of attorney.*

Alkylating agent: A type of chemotherapy drug that kills cancer cells by damaging their DNA.

Allogeneic transplant: A stem cell transplant in which the cells or tissues used come from another individual who is usually matched with the patient but not genetically identical to him or her. See also *autologous transplant.*

Alopecia: Hair loss.

Alternative therapy: A treatment that is not generally accepted as beneficial by the medical community. Often there is little or no scientific data to support use of the therapy.

Amyloidosis: A plasma cell disorder related to myeloma. It involves abnormal deposition of amyloid protein in many different organs, which can lead to dysfunction of those organs.

Analgesic: Medicine used to control or treat pain.

Ancillary therapies: Medical treatments used to prevent or relieve complications of a disease, rather than the disease itself.

Anemia: A decreased concentration of hemoglobin (the protein that transports oxygen) in the blood.

Anesthetic: Medication used to numb feeling (usually in order to perform a procedure).

Antibody: A protein that is normally produced by the body's immune system to help fight infections. Each antibody usually has a specific target that it binds to and helps to eliminate. Normally many different types (specificities) of antibodies are made, targeting different microbes. In myeloma, an excess of one or a few antibodies is produced. Also called immunoglobulin.

Aspiration: Removal of fluid from a part of the body by suction, using a needle and syringe.

Autologous transplant: A stem cell transplant in which the cells or tissues administered are derived from the patient (rather than from another individual). The term "transplant" is widely used for this procedure but is a misnomer, as nothing is being transplanted. Instead, the patient's own stem cells are collected before administration of high-dose chemotherapy. These cells are reinfused into the patient after the chemotherapy is completed. A more accurate term for this procedure is "autologous stem cell support." See also *allogeneic transplant*.

B-cells (B-lymphocyte): A type of immune cell in the body whose function is to develop into a plasma cell that produces antibodies.

Beta-2 microglobulin level: A protein that whose levels in blood indicate how much myeloma is present in the body. Its level is an indicator of prognosis.

Biologic agent: A drug that alters biological pathways in cells in order to suppress cancer.

Biopsy: Removal of a small sample of tissue for analysis under the microscope and for other testing.

Bisophosphonates: Drugs used to prevent and treat bone disease caused by myeloma.

Bone marrow: A semiliquid fatty substance contained in the cavities of bones. Blood cells are manufactured here.

Bone marrow biopsy: A diagnostic procedure in which a small amount of bone marrow fluid and/or bone is removed for examination under the microscope and other tests.

Bone marrow transplant: Aspiration of bone marrow fluid followed by infusion of the marrow into a patient. The source of the marrow can be the patient or a healthy individual.

Cancer: The uncontrolled growth of cells derived from one part of the body. Many different types of cancer exist. The more aggressive forms typically invade other tissues and grow rapidly.

Catheter: A device that provides access to either the bloodstream or a body cavity. A blood catheter is often referred to as a line.

Cell: The basic structural unit of life from which all tissues are built.

Central venous catheter: A catheter placed into one of the body's large central veins (such as the large veins in the neck or shoulder region).

Chemistry profile: A test that measures the levels of various chemicals in the blood.

Chemotherapy: The treatment of cancer using drugs or chemicals. The term is usually used to refer more specifically to drugs or chemicals that preferentially kill dividing cells.

Chromosomes: Units into which the cell's DNA is organized. Human cells typically contain 23 pairs of chromosomes each. In cancer cells the structure and number of chromosomes can be abnormal.

Clinical trial: A research study designed to assess the effectiveness and/or safety of a newer or different treatment compared to the current standard of care. This is the method whereby advances in cancer treatment occur.

Complementary therapy: Treatment used in addition to or in conjunction with standard treatments.

Complete blood count (CBC): A laboratory test that measures the number of red cells, white cells, and platelet cells in the blood and also measures the concentration of hemoglobin.

Complete remission/response (CR): Disappearance of all visible cancer from the patient's body.

Corticosteroids: Drugs chemically related to normal body hormones that control metabolism and inflammation.

Cycle (of treatment): A defined treatment period that is repeated several times in order to complete the course of therapy.

Cytogenetic analysis: A technique used to visualize chromosomes in cells and thus detect whether abnormalities are present.

DNA (deoxyribonucleic acid): The material that makes up the genetic code of most living things.

DNR order: "do not resuscitate" is a formal order written in a patient's medical chart indicating that at the patient's or family's request, acute measures to keep the patient alive will not be started.

Donor lymphocyte infusion (DLI): Administration of additional donor cells to a patient some time after an allogeneic transplant. Usually no additional preparative treatment is administered prior to the infusion of these cells.

Durable power of attorney: A legal document that entitles another person to make financial and medical decisions in case the patient becomes incapacitated. See also *advance directive*.

Flow cytometry: A test performed on blood or bone marrow that detects the amount and types of proteins that are present on or in cells.

Freelite test: A diagnostic test that measures free light chains (protein components) in the blood or urine.

Graft-versus-host disease (GVHD): A complication of allogeneic stem cell transplantation that results from an immune attack against the normal organs of the patient.

Heavy chain: Part of the biochemical structure of the antibody molecule.

Hematologist: A physician specializing in disorders of the blood (including blood and marrow cancers).

Hematopoietic: Having to do with the production of blood cells.

ImiD: Immunomodulatory molecule. Refers to compounds related to thalidomide that may stimulate the immune response against cancer in addition to other activities. .

Immunoglobulin: See *antibody*.

Immune therapy: Use of the immune system of the body to fight disease.

Immunotherapy: A type of treatment that uses the body's immune system to fight disease.

Indolent multiple myeloma (IMM): Similar to SMM, though patients with IMM may have mild anemia or a few bone lesions.

Induction therapy: Initial phase of treatment, which attempts to decrease the number of disease cells in order to relieve symptoms and prevent complications.

Kyphoplasty: A procedure to treat the pain of spinal compression fractures by injection of cement-like substance into the bone.

Lactate dehydrogenase: An enzyme protein normally found inside cells, high levels of which in the blood have been associated with a worse prognosis in several cancers.

Leukapheresis: A procedure in which blood is made to flow through a machine that skims off certain cells (usually on the basis of density) while returning everything else to the body. It is commonly used for collecting stem cells.

Leukopenia: Low white blood cell count.

Light chain: Part of the biochemical structure of the antibody molecule.

Living will: A document specifying an individual's treatment wishes in the event that he or she is unable to decide these questions.

Lytic lesions: Areas of bone thinning caused by myeloma and visible on an x-ray.

M-protein: Also known as "paraprotein," excess antibody of one type that is produced in individuals with myeloma.

Magnetic resonance imaging (MRI): A type of imaging of the inside of the body that relies on placing the patient in a strong magnetic field and detecting the changes caused in the tissues by that magnetic field.

Matched sibling donors: A transplant donor who is a full brother or sister who matches the patient for tissue type.

Matched unrelated donor: An unrelated transplant donor who is matched with the patient for tissue type.

Medical power of attorney: A document that designates an individual who will make healthcare decisions on behalf of someone who is unable to do this for himself.

Mobilization (of stem cells): The process whereby stem cells that normally reside in the bone marrow are induced to migrate into the blood temporarily, where they circulate and can be collected (harvested) for a subsequent transplant.

Monoclonal: Arising from a single clone of abnormal cells. A clone means a population of identical cells, usually arising from the division of a single cell.

Monoclonal gammopathy of undetermined significance (MGUS): A plasma cell disorder in which an abnormal monoclonal protein is produced, but that does not meet the criteria for a diagnosis of myeloma.

Multiple myeloma: A cancer of plasma cells usually arising in the bone marrow. Its features may include bone destruction, increased risk of infections, and kidney failure.

Neutropenia: An abnormally low concentration of neutrophils in the blood.

Neutrophil: The main type of white cell in the blood that fights against bacterial and fungal infections.

Oncologist: A physician specializing in the treatment of cancer. A medical oncologist specializes in the administration of chemotherapy and other drugs for the treatment of cancer.

Pathological fracture: A fracture that occurs in a bone that is weakened by a disease process. The fracture typically occurs following no trauma or minimal trauma that would be insufficient to cause a fracture in a normal bone.

Performance status: A score used by physicians to measure how well a patient can cope with the activities of daily living.

Peripheral blood stem cell transplant: A procedure like bone marrow transplantation that uses stem cells derived from blod rather than marrow.

Peripheral nervous system: Nerves that run from the brain and spinal cord to the rest of the body.

Peripheral neuropathy: Disease of or damage to nerves outside the central nervous system (brain and spinal cord). Peripheral neuropathy can be sensory (causing numbness and pain) or motor (causing weakness or paralysis) or a mix of the two.

Phase: An indication of the type of clinical trial being performed. Phase I studies are among the earliest types of clinical trial. They are conducted using a new therapy and usually need only a small number of patients. Phase III trials are large, randomized comparisons of a new therapy against the current standard of care.

Phase I trial: Early study of a treatment designed to find best dose to use and assess initial side-effects in patients.

Phase II trial: A study of a treatment already shown to be relatively safe, designed to determine its activity against the disease.

Phase III trial: A large clinical trial formally comparing a new therapy against the best standard treatment available.

Plasma cell: The type of cell that makes antibodies. It is usually produced by maturation of B-lymphocytes and is found in the bone marrow.

Plasma cell labeling index (PCLI): A test used to measure the rate of growth of myeloma cells.

Plasma cell leukemia: A type of advanced myeloma in which the abnormal plasma cells leave the bone marrow and circulate in the peripheral blood.

Plasmablastic myeloma: An aggressive type of myeloma characterized by rapid growth of the abnormal cells and an elevated LDH level.

Plasmacytoma: A localized collection of abnormal (usually monoclonal) plasma cells.

Plateau phase: A situation in which further cycles of treatment do not produce additional improvement.

Platelet: A type of cell in the blood that assists with blood clotting.

Primary amyloidosis: A disorder where insolvable protein fibers are deposited in tissues and organs, impairing their function.

Polyclonal: Arising from the division of many different cells.

Preclinical: Experimental use of a drug in animals or test-tubes, before trials in humans are conducted.

Primary Amyliodosis: A disorder related to myeloma, characterized by impaired function of many organs resulting from deposition of an abnormal protein (M-protein) in tissues.

Prognosis: A prediction of the course of the patient's disease and the patient's future prospects.

Proteasome inhibitors: A completely new class of biologic agent that act by inhibiting the proteasome—a mechanism by which cell proteins are eliminated from cells.

QIG: A diagnostic test that measures levels of the different immunoglobulin subtypes in the blood.

Radiation therapy: Treatment of cancer using x-rays or electron beam therapy.

Randomized trial: A clinical trial in which a proportion of patients get a new treatment and the remainder get the standard treatment by random assignment (that is, neither the patient nor the doctor gets to decide which of these treatments the patient will receive).

Remission: Regression of the patient's disease, with an accompanying improvement in symptoms.

SIFE: A diagnostic test that identifies the exact subtype of abnormal immunoglobulin (M-protein) produced by the myeloma.

Skeletal survey: A test in which x-rays of most of the bones of the body are taken in order to detect lytic lesions.

Smoldering multiple myeloma (SMM): A condition in which the criteria for a diagnosis of myeloma are met but the patient is in an early stage of the disease, with no symptoms.

SPEP (serum protein electrophoresis): A biochemical technique that separates and visualizes different proteins found in blood serum by running them on a gel under an electric current.

Spinal cord compression: Compression of the spinal cord (usually by a tumor or a spinal fracture), resulting in neurological symptoms. This is a medical emergency requiring rapid intervention to prevent long-term paralysis.

Stage: A means of quantifying how advanced a patient's cancer is. A higher stage number usually means that the patient has a larger bulk of cancer cells, and that they are more widespread. The Durie-Salmon staging system is the most commonly used system for staging myeloma.

Standard of care: A term used to describe the best current option for treating a disease, based upon the results of previous clinical trials.

Stem cell: A relatively nonspecialized type of cell that can generate many different types of specialized cells through division and maturation.

Support group: A group of patients with the same or similar disease offering the opportunity to share information and experience with others.

T-lymphocyte: A type of immune cell that is important in fighting viruses and cancer. It also assists other parts of the immune system.

Thrombocytopenia: Low blood platelet count.

Vaccine: An injection of a material given in order to stimulate an immune response against it.

Vertebroplasty: A procedure in which a cementlike substance is injected into a collapsed spinal bone in order to re-expand it and thus relieve pain and loss of height.

Vesicant: A type of drug that causes severe tissue damage if it leaks out from the veins into the tissues surrounding it.

Waldenstrom's disease: Sometimes referred to as Waldenstrom's macro-globulinemia. A plasma cell cancer that can be distinguished from myeloma by the production of abnormal IgM protein in the blood, which can cause increased blood viscosity. Bone destruction is usually absent.

X-ray skeletal survey: A procedure in which x-rays of all the bones in the body are taken to identify bone abnormalities caused by myeloma.

Index

Index

G

Gabapentin (Neurontin), 79
Gender differences, in myeloma development, 10
Genetic predisposition, in myeloma development, 10
Glucocorticoids. *See* Corticosteroids
Graft-versus-host-disease (GVHD), 94–97
Granulocytes, 74
Groshong catheter, 65
Growth factor drugs, 69, 75
GVHD (graft-versus-host-disease), 94–97

H

Hair loss, 72
HDC-ASCS (high-dose chemotherapy and autologous stem cell support), 43, 44
Health benefits, employer, 109–110, 117–118
Health care costs, 117–118
Health care insurance. *See* Insurance
Heavy chains, 7–8
Hematopoietic stem cells. *See* Stem cells, hematopoietic
Hemoglobin, 23, 24, 72, 76
Herbal supplements, 112–113
"Heroic" measures, 104
Hickman catheter, 65, 66
High-dose chemotherapy and autologous stem cell support (HDC-ASCS), 43, 44
HLA-identical sibling donors, 96–97, 98
Home care, 81
Hormonal treatment, for appetite stimulation, 113
Hospice, 103–104
Hospital bills, mistakes on, 118–119
Hypogammaglobulinemia, 9–10

I

IBMTR (International Bone Marrow Transplant Registry), 125
IgA
    disease progression and, 8
    in myeloma, 16, 24
    physical properties/distribution, 7
    for treatment monitoring, 67
IgD, 7, 16
IgE, 7
IgG
    disease progression and, 8
    in myeloma, 14, 16, 24

physical properties/distribution, 7
for treatment monitoring, 67
IgM, 7, 14, 16
Iliac crest, 18
ImiDs (immunomodulatory drugs), 56–57, 69
IMM (indolent multiple myeloma), 24–25, 26, 40
Immune cells, donor, 95
Immune-suppression medications, 94
Immune system
    allogeneic transplants and, 49–50
    cells of, 9. *See also specific immune system cells*
    complications, after allogeneic transplant, 93–94
    suppression, for mini transplant, 91–92
    thalidomide and, 54
    treatment effects on, 10
Immune therapy, 86–87
Immunoglobulins, 2
    abnormal, 27
    antibodies, 2, 3, 7–8
    assessment in urine, 17–18
    blood levels, in myeloma, 14
    classes, 7. *See also specific immunoglobulin classes*
    normal production, 8
    reduced levels, 27
    replacement therapy, 10, 108
    suppression of normal production, 9
    variable region of, 8
Immunomodulatory drugs (ImiDs), 56–57, 69
Immunotherapy, 41
Implantable port, 65
Incidence, of multiple myeloma, 31
Indolent multiple myeloma (IMM), 24–25, 26, 40
Induction therapy, 42
Infections
    anemia and, 76
    of catheter site, 66
    recurrent, 108
    risk of, 3, 27, 75, 93
    susceptibility to, 9–10, 73
    symptoms of, 75
Information resources, 123–126
Institutional review board, 46
Insurance
    denial of treatment, 119
    explanation of benefits, 118–119
    federally-run programs, 120
    home care and, 81
    lack of coverage, 119–121